THE
TAO *of* FERTILITY

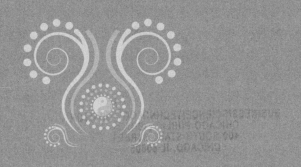

THE
TAO *of* FERTILITY

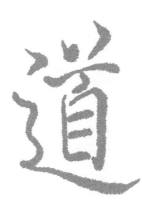

A Healing Chinese

Medicine Program to

Prepare Body, Mind,

and Spirit for New Life

Daoshing Ni, D.O.M, L.Ac., Ph.D.

and Dana Herko

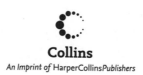

Collins
An Imprint of HarperCollinsPublishers

This book is intended to be informational and should not be considered a substitute for advice from a medical professional, whom the reader should consult before beginning any diet or exercise regimen, and before taking any dietary supplements or other medications. The author and publisher expressly disclaim responsibility for any adverse effects arising from the use or application of the information contained in this book.

The names and identifying characteristics of individuals featured throughout this book have been changed to protect their privacy.

HarperCollins books may be purchased for educational, business, or sales promotional use. For information, please write: Special Markets Department, HarperCollins Publishers, 10 East 53rd Street, New York, NY 10022.

FIRST EDITION

Designed by Nicola Ferguson
Interior illustrations by Robert Graham

Library of Congress Cataloging-in-Publication Data

Ni, Daoshing.
  The tao of fertility / Daoshing Ni and Dana Herko.—1st ed.
      p. cm.
  Includes bibliographical references and index.
  ISBN 978-0-06-113785-3
  1. Infertility, Female—Alternative treatment.   2. Medicine, Chinese.
I. Herko, Dana.   II. Title.
  RG201.N5 2008
  618.1'78—dc22   2007050400

08 09 10 RRD 10 9 8 7 6 5 4 3 2 1

To Sum Yee, Yu Ming, and Yu Chien and to my parents,
Hua-Ching Ni and Lily Chuang

To Ted, Mila, and Nick and to my parents,
Wladzia and Nicholas Herko

For teaching us the profundity of love.

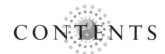

CONTENTS

CONTENTS

ACKNOWLEDGMENTS

We gratefully acknowledge all those who helped us on our journey in making this book a reality. To Toni Sciarra, our wonderful editor at HarperCollins who guided us along the path with wisdom, understanding, and encouragement—we truly couldn't have done it without you. Thank you to Nicola Ferguson for her elegant design, and to all the HarperCollins marketing, production, and publicity people who gave their time and expertise. To Robert Graham for providing us with beautiful illustrations, and to Hua Ching Ni, whose words resonate throughout this book. To Maoshing Ni, for his support and his expert suggestions, and to the doctors at the Tao of Wellness, especially Jessica Chen and James Evans, as well as Amy LeSage and Sharon Skok. To Richard Marrs and Guy Ringler for their unwavering support of Chinese medicine. To Rupert and Wendi Murdoch for believing in this project. To Ted Frank and Sum Yee Wang, our spouses: No words can convey how much your love and support mean. Most of all, to those women who so generously shared their stories and experiences: You are truly the heart of this book.

PROLOGUE

From Dr. Dao:

As a male health care professional working in traditional Chinese medicine with an emphasis on fertility, I have had the privilege of seeing thousands of women patients. I have learned a lot from them. They have taught me humility, compassion, and the strength of the human spirit. But for all I have learned—and regardless of how well I have come to appreciate and understand women—I can never be a woman living through the actual experience of her fertility challenges. I needed a woman's voice to help me better communicate the wisdom passed on to me and what I have come to know. I am fortunate to have Dana as my coauthor, who has had personal experience with the struggles of infertility and who can communicate this material with special sensitivity and awareness.

From Dana:

I first met Dr. Dao over ten years ago. I was sitting in the back row of a Santa Monica hotel ballroom packed with hundreds of other women who were trying to have a baby. My friend Ellen was with me; like me, she had married in her thirties and was finding that getting pregnant wasn't as easy as we'd been led to believe. The conference was sponsored by RESOLVE, a nonprofit organization dedicated to helping women deal with fertility and adoption issues. One of the speakers was a doctor who spoke about the advances in reproductive technology; another was an advocate for domestic adoption; yet another talked about foreign adoptions and foster children. The final speaker was a Chinese medical doctor. He spoke about acupuncture and holistic medicine and how getting healthy could help women improve their fertility.

Frankly, my friend and I weren't terribly interested. Adoption, fertility drugs, in vitro fertilization (IVF)—these seemed like sure things—maybe not immediate, maybe expensive, but guarantees of having children. Chinese medicine sounded so . . . basic. Yes, it was good to be health-minded, but it seemed like a long road to take when all these other options were available and the clock was ticking.

Little did I know.

Three years later, after a few stalled adoption attempts, multiple rounds of IVF, and several miscarriages, I found myself sitting in the office of yet another fertility doctor—fortunately, one whose expertise in assisted reproductive medicine was matched by his compassion. He slid a small business card across the desk and said, "His name is Dr. Dao. I don't know exactly how it works or even why. But it might just help if you're willing to believe . . ."

Willing to believe. At that point, I was willing to believe in anything that would result in a real, live baby. The African fertility god sculpture sent by a well-meaning friend, the St. Anthony medal from my church back in New York, the little artifact from Lourdes . . . I was armed and ready for a miracle. But Chinese medicine? What seemed like a long road back in that Santa Monica hotel now looked like an impossible detour. I wasn't sure I was ready to make that journey because, to put it bluntly, I was worn down and flat-out exhausted from trying to get pregnant. I was nearing forty with nothing to show for my efforts except a growing pile of bills for examinations, fertility drugs, specialists, hospital stays, sonograms, and endless blood tests to see if anything—let alone, anyone—was growing inside of me.

Most of all, I was tired of doctors. I had naively thought that when it came time to get pregnant and have a baby, one doctor did it all. I wasn't prepared for the stream of specialists who poked, prodded, and pronounced judgment each time another pregnancy attempt failed. It was my uterus; no, it was my blood; it was my age; no, it was my immune system; it was my tubes; it was my pelvis . . . it was, as it turned out, simply unexplained. But each doctor had a theory, and perhaps each doctor was even right. The trouble was, they were all looking at my parts. None of them were looking at me as a whole person. Having grown up with Western medicine, it wasn't odd, just frustrating. It was simply the way things were.

One day, while waiting in yet another doctor's office for results of yet another test, a childhood rhyme suddenly came back to me: " 'I see,' said the blind man. 'The elephant is very like a tree!' " All these blind men, picking at different parts of the elephant, each one getting a different picture of what the elephant was—a tree if he touched the trunk, a snake if he held the tail; none of them wrong, but none of them entirely right. And there I was—the elephant. No wonder I was skeptical when the fertility specialist suggested Dr. Dao. Did I really need another blind man?

I talked to my husband about trying Chinese medicine, but I didn't tell anyone else. Very few of even my closest friends and family knew I was going through fertility treatments, because unlike other medical conditions, infertility can seem almost elective—at least to women who never struggled to have children. Break a leg, wear a cast, and everyone will ask you about it. Break your heart by losing another child through miscarriage, and even the kindest people run out of things to say. So you just stop talking about your attempts to have children even though it means having to hear the well-intentioned cautions not to wait too long and reminders that your career might be important, but you aren't getting any younger.

Some people told me to simply relax and that a baby would come naturally. Meanwhile, I had become an expert in chemistry. I knew just when I had to take fertility drugs each month, which pharmacy carried them, how many vials to use, how to mix the powders with the solutions, and what size needle to use. As a child, I used to get sick at the sight of needles. Now I was shooting up in my bathroom at least twice a day at rigidly appointed times. I would go to the lab the first thing in the morning for a blood test, then spend the day waiting for the call from the nurse giving me the exact drug dosage I needed that night—me, someone who doesn't even use a measuring cup when I cook.

The first time I attempted IVF, I wouldn't go out at night in case I had to give myself an injection. Only once did I risk it, which is how I found myself with a needle in a stall in the ladies' room of the local movie theater during an early evening showing of *Gosford Park*. By the second year, I had become so good at giving myself injections that two fellow fertility travelers whose husbands were out of town asked me to give them their shots. But silence, not sisterhood, was the norm. I learned—or at least tried—to decompartmentalize infertility and make it just another part of my life, along with marriage, family, friends, and work.

Most of the women interviewed for this book were working full-time jobs while trying to get pregnant, and the majority of them hid the fact from their employers and coworkers. I know I did, which was often difficult since I was writing for a soap opera on the opposite coast. Because of the three-hour time difference, conference calls that typically lasted all day began at 6:00 A.M. my time. Unfortunately, that happened to be the exact time I was expected to show up at the lab for my daily blood tests. For three years I spent an average of three hours a day driving from my home in Hollywood to the fertility clinic in Santa Monica and back again, all the while pretending I was at my desk instead of negotiating LA rush-hour traffic.

I told myself I was lucky to have work to take my mind off my fertility attempts. But there were times when the two became uncomfortably intermingled. When one of the characters on my soap got married (for want of a better story line), I prayed we'd think of something for her over the next six months that didn't involve pregnancy. Two months later, she was not only pregnant but in the hospital fighting to save the life of her unborn child. And because I was reluctant to share that I had just had a miscarriage, guess which writer drew that story line? My life had become surreal. My rational mind told me that I couldn't handle one more fertility treatment, but my heart had a grip on me and wouldn't let go.

I made a bargain with myself: one visit to this Dr. Dao. At least then I would know that I had tried everything. I was hoping for a baby, but I was ready to settle for peace.

I stepped into Dr. Dao's waiting room and into a white light. Sunshine was everywhere. There were shelves of Chinese health books and a large urn of herbal tea. There was sound—not actually music to my Western ear, more like birds chirping in a forest. What struck me the most were the pregnant women calmly sipping tea—a sight rarely if ever seen in a fertility clinic. I had learned firsthand that women lucky enough to become and stay pregnant for three months "graduated" from the clinic to an ob-gyn. A few of the women in Dr. Dao's office looked ready to go into labor right then and there.

A pleasant woman in a white jacket ushered me into a room that looked more like a professor's study than an office. A moment later, Dr. Dao entered and gave me a big hug. Needless to say, I was completely caught off-guard. He then sat down and gently started asking questions— not just about my medical history and what brought me there (although, I suspect, the misery on my face spoke volumes) but how I was feeling emotionally. He wanted to hear everything—not just about my miscarriages but my life story from the moment I married and decided to try to get pregnant. I started slowly, then built up speed as I tried to purge myself of all my built-up grief before he cut me off. But he never did. Instead, when I finally had finished talking, Dr. Dao politely asked if he could take my pulse and have a look at my tongue. A moment later, he said he could help me.

I just stared at him. No tests? No labs? Dr. Dao explained that he had a sense of what my problem was and was confident he could help me. But it would take time, patience, and most importantly, a willingness to change the way I looked at my body and health and my very life.

I left the office thinking it was an interesting experience. But investing more time seemed pointless when I had so little time left. Dr. Dao wanted me to try acupuncture and herbal treatments for three months. I was not convinced.

The next day the phone rang. It was Dr. Dao wanting to know how I was. I thanked him for asking and waited to hear the real purpose of his call. It finally dawned on me: he simply wanted to know how I was, regardless of whether I decided to try Chinese medicine. He was checking on someone who obviously inspired concern.

I started to cry. A week later, I started treatment—an all-encompassing program that included not only acupuncture and herbs but dietary changes and stress-relief suggestions. I gave him the three months he asked for.

Those three months have turned into nine years. During that time, I have been blessed with two children I love beyond anything I could ever have imagined. So yes, I have firsthand proof that Chinese medicine can really work when other paths to fertility seem too hard to travel. I know how fortunate I am. I also know how I felt when, at my most despairing, I read yet another book about a fertility-challenged woman having a baby (and believe me, I read them all). Even though I came away with hope, a small part of me always thought, easy for her to say—she has children.

Maybe some of you are reading this with the same reaction. All I can say is that Chinese medicine and the underlying concept of Taoism have changed my life in ways far beyond helping me become a mother. They have helped me through unexpected issues after having children, and they continue to remind me that the journey—not the destination—is really the point of life. Based on the number of women I interviewed for this book, I know that I am not alone.

At one point when Dr. Dao and I first discussed writing this book, he mentioned a story from his childhood about the mythical adventures of a monkey. This Monkey King, according to Dr. Dao, was on a difficult journey. He had to overcome so many obstacles and hardships that he often thought of giving up and going home. But the Monkey King didn't because Buddha had placed a band of metal around his head. When the Monkey King wanted to quit, Buddha tightened the band. The headache was a reminder of things left undone.

My band was around my heart. Every time I thought of giving up, I tried to imagine how I would feel years later. If it turned out I was unable to have children, could I honestly tell myself that I had done all that I could? As I said, I was beyond fortunate. I found peace *and* children. May you be as blessed.

INTRODUCTION

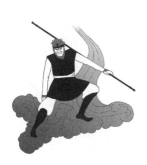

Every child in China knows the story of the Monkey King. It's an age-old parable about a monkey who is born from a rock when it splits in two. He's all-powerful, full of magic—and yes, of himself. After all, he is the Monkey King.

He amuses himself, getting into all kinds of mischief as he conquers the world. But soon, the earthly world loses its challenges, and with it, its charm. As always, the Monkey King wants more. He wants to be immortal, so he flies to Heaven to seek his immortality. There he finds the God of Heaven, having tea with his good friend, Buddha.

Being the bold little creature that he is, the Monkey King quickly takes matters into his own hands. He orders the God of Heaven to vacate his seat. Buddha, good friend that he is, realizes that the God of Heaven surely has better things to do than deal with an impudent monkey. So he intervenes and tells the Monkey King: "If you can jump out of my hand, *then* you can have the seat of the God of Heaven."

Well. Imagine for a moment how powerful the Monkey King feels now. Here is Buddha offering the God of Heaven's seat—and all the Monkey King has to do is fly to the end of the world. The Monkey King gleefully soars from Heaven. He keeps flying, all the way to the end of the world. There he finds five misty mountains that are massive and grand. The little monkey by now is so arrogant, so full of himself and his powers that it is not enough to know that he has reached the end of the universe. No, he has to leave behind proof that he has so easily done the undoable. So he pees on the mountain, to mark his territory, leave proof of his presence, and show one and all his power. After this, he is so pleased that he flies back to Heaven to confront Buddha. "See what I can do!" the Monkey King brags. Buddha looks at the creature with pity. Then he slowly opens his hand. "You might want to see what you did, little monkey." There, in Buddha's hand, is the small dampness where the Monkey King has so proudly peed.

Buddha throws the Monkey King back to Earth, where he is buried deep into a mountain with only his head protruding. And there the Monkey King stays for thousands and thousands of years until a compassionate Buddha decides to give him a chance to repent by calling him on a very special journey.

Perhaps right about now you are thinking: But what does a Chinese fairy tale about a monkey have to do with me? After all, you are trying to have a baby—that's most likely why you picked up this book. And yet, on closer look, do you not see some parallels between the Monkey King's life and your own? The Monkey King is strong-willed, knows exactly what he wants, and is brilliant at what he does. He has special powers, although he does not yet know how to use them; he plays and enjoys his life on Earth until one day a small cloud appears in his mind when he looks around and for the first time sees that all his monkey friends are aging—dying, even. "But surely that will never happen to me," the Monkey King rationalizes. "After all, I am immortal." So the cloud passes as quickly as it came, and the Monkey King does nothing. He just keeps playing and working until one day, while reaching for a higher place, he's slammed back to Earth—hard.

Maybe you are already thinking that you are going to get old one day. You sense that time is passing; as the years have gone by, you have begun to think more and more about having a baby. But not yet, you may have said to yourself. Wait until the time is right, until you meet the right partner, until you are settled in your career. You still have time; you are still young. At least you feel young, and what's more, you feel healthy. When the time is right, getting pregnant will not be a problem. How many news stories have there been about women getting pregnant in their late thirties, forties, even in their fifties? There is time; maybe not endless time, but time enough.

Women take it for granted that it's their natural right to have children. But you can only push nature so far. I first learned this lesson when

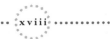

Women's Voices

"I got married at thirty-one. I was in no rush. I really didn't think about having children until two or three years later. I was working and traveling.... I liked my life. I wasn't so sure I wanted the responsibility of having children. I thought if it happens, great. Of course, I assumed it really would happen. Or that I would start thinking about it ... sometime. I took a lot for granted."

I was a little boy, growing up in Taiwan. Typhoons were a regular occurrence. The house I lived in had three stories—it was a simple but sturdy house with thin walls and windows on the third floor. Whenever a typhoon was expected, my mother would close the windows on the top floor of the house so that the wind had no chance to enter, for if a single window were left open, all the windows would be broken by the power of the storm. During a typhoon, the rule was clear: I was never to go to the third floor in case the windows did shatter, hurling glass all around.

So naturally enough, I went to the third floor. I remember listening to the wind, hearing the windows rattle and shake. That's when I first realized how potent and powerful nature is. And yet there I was, defying all odds to go against it. I came down from the third floor and slipped out of the house. Despite the howling winds and rapidly flooding streets— and my mother's strict instructions to stay indoors—I wanted to play.

Seeing scaffolding from a neighboring house under construction, I turned the wooden plank into a makeshift bridge above the rising waters. Nothing was going to deter me from my plan.

But nature had other ideas. Suddenly, a massive wind ripped a giant piece of tin awning from the unfinished house and sent it hurling directly toward me. I froze. Fortunately, the awning hit the concrete post holding up the house instead of me. I can still remember the sound of that giant *bang!* as the tin reverberated. Needless to say, I ran home as fast as I could. I fought nature, and nature fought back.

As a Taoist, I believe that nature is not always there to serve us. But from the day we are born, it's all about pushing the envelope. Everything we do is an attempt to push nature as part of our innate instinct to not only survive but thrive. We may not be meant to climb Mount Everest, but that doesn't stop people from trying. We are not meant to fly—how many of us were born with wings? Instead, we travel by jets in defiance of nature. All creatures on this earth defy nature, because life is all about push and pull. There are actions, and there are consequences.

Yes, you can wait to start a family. But it becomes increasingly difficult after the age of thirty-five. That's nature at work. Conventional medicine can help with assisted reproductive technology but not without a price. I am not just speaking in terms of financial costs but also of costs to your spirit and your well-being. We now know that drugs used to stimulate the reproductive system can trigger complications and side effects ranging from weight gain to earlier menopause, among other things. If used excessively, these fertility drugs can potentially cause your system to age much faster than it normally would.

And yet Taoist philosophy is not about looking at situations and judging what is right and what is wrong. It is about understanding how the universe works and about taking responsibility for your life and your actions. Taoism comes from observation of nature. If you look at just one day, for example, you will see certain natural rhythms. You will see the sun rise and then set; you will see day and night. There is a certainty and a pattern. But within these patterns, there is also chaos. Sometimes it is too hot in the summer. Sometimes the frost comes too early. There's rain, there's drought, there's wind. There are little changes, too. Each day is a little different from the day before—just as each day your energy changes.

One of the symbols of Taoism is tai ji, with its curved, divided halves. One half is white; the other is black. Each contains a dot of the opposing color. What that means—to us, to the world—is that nature is always trying to reach homeostasis or balance. There is no such thing as perfect balance or perfect truth in the world. There is no such thing as perfection. A curving line is always changing, always fluid. Sometimes it is blacker, and sometimes it is whiter.

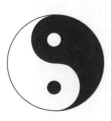

Tai ji symbol

But it is never truly balanced. The world is always living in some kind of chaos and is always trying to find some organization in that chaos.

When you are struggling to become pregnant, the important thing is not to despair. You must remember that you are both working with and fighting against nature. Fortunately, you have a powerful ally in traditional Chinese medicine.

Some people use the term *alternative* when talking about traditional Chinese medicine (TCM). But to me, there is a stigma attached to that word. It has a connotation that TCM is somehow not mainstream simply because it is not Western medicine. I prefer the term *natural*. Like Taoism, TCM is based on embracing nature and understanding the world. In Taoism, you care about improving yourself, and you always, always embrace nature rather than damage it. Taoists find the answers to life's questions in nature. This is also what TCM does.

TCM is holistic. The first principle of TCM is that every system works together. If one system breaks down, it will affect the other systems. The body is more than a collection of parts; it is an organic entity. Many different systems and organs function in an intimate fashion. When we treat a particular system, we must keep all the other systems in mind.

This brings us to the second principle of TCM: the human body's relationship with nature. Because we, as humans, are members of nature, nature provides and supplies energy to help us survive. Changes in nature will indirectly or directly change our body. Consider a huge natural disaster: a tsunami or hurricane or earthquake that causes massive destruction and creates immense death, injury, and damage. This type of unforeseen occurrence in nature will have a direct effect on our body and our health. And yet the effect will not be permanent: History tells us—and modern events bear out—that people are amazingly resilient. They overcome, they rebuild, and they forget—at least until the next disaster strikes. That is what nature is all about. It rebuilds and it recycles. It is a normal cycle of life and death.

Finally, there is the third principle of TCM: the relationship between humans and the societies they create. Humans are social beings. The way we drive, the way we speak, the way we interact, taxes, pollution . . . all affect us. People's emotions—whether joy, sadness, anger, grief, or fright—all create different imbalances in our body, which can create imbalances in our organ systems.

Chinese medicine is all about teaching women to look at the natural approach to dealing with infertility. The word *teach* is important because TCM asks that you become an authority on your own condition. Did you know that patients in China are responsible for keeping their own medical records? It's true. When you go to a doctor in China, the doctor notes your visit on the file you have brought with you. In TCM, you and your doctor are partners. Ideally, you should have some ability to understand your medical condition and start doing what you can to improve your odds of conceiving even before you seek medical help.

Growing numbers of women have helped their chances of getting pregnant and maintaining a healthy pregnancy by adhering to the tenets of TCM. I am not just talking about going to a Chinese practitioner or doctor for acupuncture. I am referring to using techniques, diets, exercise, and even over-the-counter herbs and medications known to improve the chances of pregnancy, and even more importantly, good health.

The reality is that women want to get pregnant at all costs. But the potential for success starts with making sure your body is as healthy as possible. The same goes for your emotional and spiritual state. It is the foundation for getting pregnant and for maintaining health and vitality after the baby is born.

When compared to the conventional approach to medicine, it sounds like a lot of work. And to someone used to being taken care of by doctors, it is. In many developed countries, we have basically institutionalized medicine to take care of our health. I believe that we should allow our

Women's Voices

"In Western medicine, they can tell you what they see. But they don't have to tell you what they know. It's never the complete picture. It's always some half information."

body to heal naturally, instead of surrendering control of it to a medical establishment.

Unquestionably, modern medicine has a lot to offer. Every day in my practice, I work closely with Western fertility experts. Assisted reproductive technology (ART) has helped many couples around the world to have the children of their dreams. The impact of this technology is far-reaching and profound. Research has shown that women who are undergoing ART such as IVF can increase their odds by using Chinese medicine at the same time. But I am against the principle of passively turning your well-being over to someone else. In fact, if you are sick and you go to a doctor and pop a pill, you are, in effect, placing your life entirely in someone else's hands. You aren't taking responsibility for your health—your doctor is.

Responsibility. Remember our friend the Monkey King? By failing to take responsibility for his actions, he ends up banished to the bottom of a mountain. The Monkey King has to start at square one. All that he has is taken from him. What lies ahead is a journey filled with seemingly insurmountable obstacles and an uncertain final destination. And yet, as we shall see later on, each struggle and each challenge brings enlightenment and a better understanding of himself.

All life is a journey. Fertility is life, making it the ultimate journey. Whatever road you have traveled thus far in your desire to have a child—whether just thinking about it, trying to conceive naturally, or using the tools of modern reproductive medicine such as IVF—I am asking you to begin the journey anew. Put your toes to the fire. Ask yourself: What have I done with my body? Is there any way I can enhance it, make it healthier? As in any journey, you will need to be prepared. As your partner and guide, I will provide tools to help you improve your general health and increase your awareness of your body.

No one knows what lies ahead. But isn't that the beauty of life?

THE

JOURNEY BEGINS:

Preparing Mind, Body, and Spirit

Tackle difficulties when they are easy.

Accomplish great things when they are small.

Handle what is going to be rough

When it is still smooth.

Control what has not yet formed its force.

Deal with a dangerous situation while it is still safe.

Manage what is hard while it is soft.

Eliminate what is vicious

Before it becomes destructive.

This is called

Attending to great things at small beginnings.

—FROM *THE COMPLETE WORKS OF LAO TZU,*
TRANSLATION AND ELUCIDATION BY HUA-CHING NI

FINDING YOUR FOOTING

Enjoy good health.
Weaken your ambitions.
Strengthen your essence.

—FROM *THE COMPLETE WORKS OF LAO TZU,*
TRANSLATION AND ELUCIDATION BY HUA-CHING NI

After thousands and thousands of years in exile, the Monkey King finally gets a break. Buddha summons him and tells him to get ready, for a long journey awaits him. A monk has been appointed to bring back the sacred scriptures. He will have to travel all the way from China to India and then back again, with the Monkey King as his escort.

Fortunately, the journey you are about to embark on is not quite as long, at least not when measured in miles. But the challenges you face trying to get pregnant can be every bit as daunting. You need to prepare yourself for whatever lies ahead. How can you do this when you might not even know what you are facing? You do it by making sure you are physically, emotionally, and spiritually strong before taking even a single step.

In traditional Chinese medicine, the mind, the body, and the spirit are one. You do not live your life in a vacuum. Nor do you stand still—you are in motion every second, every minute, every day of your life. Imagine a clock with the pendulum swinging. But while the pendulum is moving, so is the clock, trying to find balance in motion. Now think of your body. When you are stressed, overworked, emotional . . . guess what happens?

You leave yourself vulnerable to outside forces like viruses, germs, and bacteria. Sickness, by definition, is the imbalance of yin and yang, or interopposing and intersupporting forces.

You are a complete and complex individual with a unique constitution. What establishes being in balance for you is entirely different than balance for someone else. Our circumstances, our surroundings, our genetics all leave an imprint on us. In traditional Chinese medicine, there are no absolutes. Everything is relative. There's no such thing as perfect health. But there is better health. And better health means better fertility. You hold the power to attain it.

You could say that my family has been at this for a long time. I come from almost seventy-six generations of Taoists. Taoism is a lineage, in the same way Judaism and many other spiritual traditions are. But it's less a religion than a way of life. It is based on embracing nature and understanding the world. It teaches you to care about improving yourself. Most importantly, it teaches you to always embrace nature rather than damage it. In a way, it's not that different from what Henry David Thoreau, in *Walden Pond,* believed: that you must preserve nature at all costs. We believe this because the answers to life's questions lie in nature.

In order to try and understand the philosophical underpinnings of balance—of health and sickness, of life and death—Taoists focus on five

Women's Voices

"Don't give up until you've opened yourself up to alternatives. This is something that is holistic. Your spirit is so crushed by the process of fertility, and Dao raises up your spirit in a human way. He thinks of you as a person and not just a baby machine. This is part of what he offers—a way of treating the whole person. He gives you a realistic picture in a very ancient but modern way. He allowed me to go on with my life when I was in my deepest despair."

major areas of study. A child growing up as I did in the Taoist tradition chooses early on which of these paths to walk. There's astrology, as in fortune-telling, which teaches how constellations and human energies affect out lives. I Ching is another form of fortune-telling, but one based on randomness. It teaches how to handle and manage changes in our lives. Another path is feng shui, the study of how the placement of objects affects our energy and how our physical environment can be conducive to our life force. There's martial arts, which teaches how to find inspiration and knowledge in the observation of animal movement in nature—a knowledge that can then be used to strengthen our body and increase our understanding of the relationships among people. And finally, there is healing.

I was predestined to be a healer. I started on this path when I was just a little boy. But I did not start with the study of medicine or healing, because for Taoists, the five paths are just extensions of life itself. My father and mother taught me first and above all how to be a good person. That is the Taoist way. We started with an understanding of the good and the bad in the universe, and learned how life worked. My brother— who is also a healer—and I learned to sweep floors, to help out, to understand the importance of family and the social unit. We also learned the importance of cultivating yourself and taking personal responsibility. Many people hear the word *responsibility* and think of some heavy burden. But as a child, my responsibility was to play hard and study hard, and to appreciate the life I was given. That's all I was asked to do.

Yet even as I went about my everyday life of playing and doing simple chores, I was learning profound lessons. Take a little thing like sweeping the floor. Looking back, I see that sweeping was so much more than cleaning. It was the way I swept the floor: the patterns I created, the way I felt when I was doing the task. Every day, there was a different energy to my sweeping. Some days, I felt impatient. Other days, I felt so good that I did a little extra work. And on those days when I felt particularly happy, I could see things I wouldn't have noticed otherwise, like the dust particles on the hardwood floor and the way they danced in the light.

By the time I was in elementary school, I started learning tai chi chuan and chi gong, two Taoist forms of meditative exercise that require

Women's Voices

"There are so few people who really love what they do—and he [Dr. Dao] does. You can read it on his face. But I don't know if he understands how much he empowers the women he sees."

contemplative thinking and silence. At the time, I didn't understand this silence and why the people were standing like statues. But slowly I could see the value of this kind of quiet time and the lessons you could learn from it. It taught me how to be calm. That was the real beginning of becoming a healer. I was learning the Taoist ways that would prepare me to go on and learn the practice of Chinese medicine.

So what is Taoism? As I've mentioned, it's the philosophy that you are one hundred percent responsible for your behavior. You *are* your own behavior; your actions are a reflection of your energy. Above all, Taoism means looking beyond your immediate world. If, for example, safety and prosperity are provided to me, I, in turn, give back more to the world to make it a more peaceful place. As a healer, one of the ways I can do that is to help people actualize their life and their potential. If your goal is motherhood, my role is to serve as your guide along the way.

I am thankful for what I have. I must embrace whatever life dishes out. And I must do so without prejudice, without blame, and without frustration. That is what the Taoist tradition teaches me. Life is a process, a journey of many different destinations. So come, let us begin.

The Importance of Good Nutrition

Have you ever seen a beautiful flower growing in concrete? Most likely, you have not. A flower needs more than the sun and water to grow. It needs nourishment. It cannot thrive in rocks and dry dirt. If it doesn't get the right mix of soil and nutrients, it will wither and eventually die.

Like that flower, you need good nutrition in order to maintain good health and to ensure your fertility. The best way to good nutrition is through food. Obviously, there are situations where you might use supplements and vitamins. But if you are relying on them as your main focus, you are wrong. Eating healthy foods should be your primary concern. Your body absorbs nutrients the best from whole foods. Taoists have a particular perspective when it comes to food. In the United States, we tend to talk about food in terms of the form it takes. Is it fast food? Organic? Natural? Processed? Prepared? But food is like everything else in the Taoist tradition: it's all about harmony and balance—yin and yang.

Growing up, I ate the food my mother prepared. It wasn't until I began to learn Taoist and traditional Chinese medicine that I realized her cooking and food preparation have always been based on the yin-and-yang principle, which takes into consideration both the energetic qualities and the taste of food.

All foods—and for that matter, herbs—have five tastes. The sweet taste is nourishing and calming. If you have ever suffered from PMS and craved sweets, then you know what I am talking about. Sweet foods can calm and quiet down the nervous system when inner stress strikes. The sour taste is astringent and consolidating. Berries, oranges, and vinegars are a few examples of sour foods. They are very good at holding up the body, especially when it is fatigued. The third taste, pungent, is dispersing and moving. Spicy foods fall into this group. They are good at warming the body by moving our circulation. The fourth taste is bitter. The body craves bitter foods like coffee or tea when it needs an energy or mood pickup, or when it needs to feel cleansed. And finally, there is the salty taste. Think of meat tenderizers—they soften the meat. So salt relaxes and softens the body.

In addition, all foods carry one of four qualities. Foods are hot (to invigorate and heat up the body), warm (to gently warm the body), cool (to gently cool the body), or cold (to vigorously cleanse the body). It's all a matter of common sense, really. When you are chilled in the winter, you need foods like hot soup, beef, or lamb. If, however, you are running a fever and need to be cooled down, pears, watermelon, and water can help.

The Chinese believe that the end result of observing these food qualities and then combining them in a harmonious manner is good health and a sense of well-being. There's nothing mysterious or complicated about it. It's another way of saying that you should be mindful of what you eat, and of when and why you are eating it. As we shall see, these things are greatly important when you are eating to improve your fertility.

In my practice, I see many women for whom weight is an issue. More often than not, they are looking for a way to shed pounds quickly, even while they are pursuing their goal of motherhood. It is true that carrying excess weight on your frame is not the ideal start to a pregnancy. But it is just as true that women who carry too little weight can face difficulties in becoming and staying pregnant. As with everything else in Chinese medicine, the underlying concept is balance.

You cannot go on a restrictive diet. That applies anytime, especially when you are trying to enhance your fertility. It doesn't matter if the diet is high protein, or high fat, or low carbohydrate. The only diet you should be following during this critical time before motherhood is a balanced one. Any diet that doesn't include the major food groups is not healthy for fertility.

But what if you don't eat meat? If you are a vegetarian for philosophical reasons, I will be frank: you will be lacking certain nutrients that you can't get from eating plants alone. You can, however, supplement your diet by taking B complex, specifically B12 and B6. B complex is a blend of a group of eight B vitamins: vitamin B1 (thiamine), vitamin B2 (riboflavin), vitamin B3 (niacin), vitamin B5 (pantothenic acid), vitamin B6 (pyridoxine and pyridoxamine), vitamin B7 (biotin), vitamin B9 (folic acid), and vitamin B12 (cyanocobalamin). Of these, the most important for fertility health are B12, B6, and B9. Vitamin B9 is especially critical, both before and during the first months of your pregnancy. Folic acid helps the fetus to develop normally, especially the neural tubes. The risk of malformations of the spine (spina bifida), skull, and brain (anencephaly) is drastically reduced when you take supplemental folic acid. The recommended dietary allowance (RDA) of folic acid supplements for pregnant women is 600 micrograms daily. This is especially important if you are over the age of thirty-five.

You should incorporate more protein in your diet however you can. Vegetarism shouldn't just be about avoiding meat. You must follow such a diet mindfully and carefully.

Chinese medicine treats everyone individually. No two women are exactly the same size or build. When you are embarking on the path to fertility, it is important that your body be in balance. That includes carrying the proper amount of body fat and weight for your particular frame. Having too little body fat can be just as detrimental as having too much. If you have any doubts, there are certain guidelines that can help you decide whether your weight is in balance for your height and body type. One of the most helpful tools is the body mass index (BMI).

The BMI is a number derived from a calculation of your weight and height. By accurately indicating your percentage of body fat, it helps identify weight categories that may or may not lead to health problems. It is calculated by dividing your weight in pounds by your height in inches squared and then multiplying that sum by 703. For example, if you weigh 150 pounds and are 5'5" (or 65"), the calculation would be:

$$(150 \div 65^2) \times 703 = 24.96$$

Or a simpler way would be to look at the table on the next page. Find your height as indicated in the column on the left, then find the point where your weight in pounds intersects your height. Trace that point to the top row, which is where you can find your approximate BMI. For example, if your height is 5'5" (65") and your weight is 146 pounds, your BMI falls between 24 and 25 kg/m². Using the BMI number you have found in the top row, look at the table to find your weight status. Following our earlier example, a BMI between 24 and 25 kg/m² would put you at the borderline of the overweight category.

Just as important as how much you weigh is how you eat. Women who come to my practice often admit their eating habits aren't the best. They want to change the way they eat and like the idea of cleansing their body first so that they can start from the ground up. That is why I've included the following eating plan. It's a one-week specialized plan specifically designed for detoxification. It is a good way to jump-start your body into becoming healthier and to introduce your mind to a leaner way of eating. It's also very good if you find yourself taking fertility drugs at some point in your fertility journey (for example, in between rounds of artificial insemination or IVF procedures) and want to rebalance your system after their use. The only

BMI (KG/ M²)	19	20	21	22	23	24	25	26	27	28	29	30	35	40
HEIGHT (IN.)	WEIGHT (LB.)													
58	91	96	100	105	110	115	119	124	129	134	138	143	167	191
59	94	99	104	109	114	119	124	128	133	138	143	148	173	198
60	97	102	107	112	118	123	128	133	138	143	148	153	179	204
61	100	106	111	116	122	127	132	137	143	148	153	158	185	211
62	104	109	115	120	126	131	136	142	147	153	158	164	191	218
63	107	113	118	124	130	135	141	146	152	158	163	169	197	225
64	110	116	122	128	134	140	145	151	157	163	169	174	204	232
65	114	120	126	132	138	144	150	156	162	168	174	180	210	240
66	118	124	130	136	142	148	155	161	167	173	179	186	216	247
67	121	127	134	140	146	153	159	166	172	178	185	191	223	255
68	125	131	138	144	151	158	164	171	177	184	190	197	230	262
69	128	135	142	149	155	162	169	176	182	189	196	203	236	270
70	132	139	146	153	160	167	174	181	188	195	202	207	243	278
71	136	143	150	157	165	172	179	186	193	200	208	215	250	286
72	140	147	154	162	169	177	184	191	199	206	213	221	258	294
73	144	151	159	166	174	182	189	197	204	212	219	227	265	302
74	148	155	163	171	179	186	194	202	210	218	225	233	272	311
75	152	160	168	176	184	192	200	208	216	224	232	240	279	319
76	156	164	172	180	189	197	205	213	221	230	238	246	287	328

BMI	WEIGHT STATUS
Below 18.5	Underweight
18.5–24.9	Normal
25.0–29.9	Overweight
30.0 and Above	Obese
Source: Centers for Disease Control, Department of Health and Human Services, http://www.cdc.gov/nccdphp/dnpa/bmi/ index.htm.	

thing I would warn is not to undertake the program if you are already normal or underweight, with a body fat level below 25.

The program used in my clinic is easy to follow, with foods that are readily available. Basically you will be consuming vegetables, grains, and protein (chicken, turkey, or soy). In addition, you will need to take supplements that are explained in more detail at the end of the diet.

Tao of Wellness One-Week Detox Diet

Upon Rising
Acidophilus or probiotic supplement (see Probiotic Supplement, page *14)*
Lemon water (the juice of one lemon squeezed in 12 ounces of filtered
    water. The water should be room temperature.

This is slightly acidic; it helps to cleanse and move the roughage that stays behind in your intestines and your system, especially when taken on an empty stomach.

Breakfast
Brown rice with soy milk
    or
Oat bran cereal with soy milk

The amount depends on the size of your body. But the best range is 4 to 8 ounces of cooked rice or oat bran. The brown rice should be organic; so should the soy milk. Use unsweetened soy milk, without added flavor or sugar. You can mix a cup of the soy milk—8 ounces—into the rice or oat bran, or drink it alone. All Bran cereal is fine; so is any other whole grain cereal as long as it is unbleached and does not contain added sugar or chemicals.

Detox tea (8 ounces)

Ideally, this is herbal tea prescribed by your practitioner. But there are many good substitutes easily found in most health food stores. Some good ones include:

Green tea (strong antioxidant)
Sarsaparilla root (gas and urine cleanser)

Milk thistle seeds (gallbladder, liver, and spleen cleanser)

Red clover (blood purifier)

Dandelion root (liver cleanser)

Yellow dock root (liver cleanser)

Burdock root (liver and urine cleanser)

Hibiscus flower (stomach cleanser)

Echinacea angustifolia flower (lymphatic system cleanser)

Fenugreek seed (lung support and cleanser)

Ginger root (bowel and kidney cleanser)

Cascara sagrada bark (liver, gallbladder, pancreas, and stomach cleanser)

Midmorning Snack

8 ounces of vegetable juice and 8 ounces of vegetable broth

You can make your own *vegetable juice* by juicing the following together: cabbage; cucumber; carrots (including greens); celery; turnips; asparagus; beets (including greens); parsley; apple; aloe vera (can be found in liquid form in most health food stores); 1 slice fresh ginger root.

You can just as easily buy a bottle of vegetable juice from the supermarket or health food store. Just make sure to read the label to ensure that it contains no added salt or chemicals. Don't be fooled by the word *natural* on the label. If there are synthetic additives in it, don't drink it.

To make *vegetable broth*, add as many of the following as you can in a large pot of filtered water: collards; Swiss chard; kale; mustard greens; dandelion; brussels sprouts; daikon radish; watercress; seaweed (any type); shiitake mushroom; cilantro; garlic; leeks; fennel (¼ teaspoon, preferably fresh); anise (1–2 pieces); ginger (3 slices); turmeric (¼ teaspoon). Boil until all ingredients are soft; strain. (*Note:* This broth can be made in larger batches and refrigerated for two or three days.)

Lunch and Dinner

For each meal, choose one of the following options. (*Note:* You can change options daily, or stick with the choice you like. Whenever possible, organic items are preferred. Chicken, turkey, fish, or soy products can be grilled, steamed, baked, or sautéed in water or in a tablespoon of walnut oil—in fact, prepared in any way except for deep-fried. Vegetables can be steamed or sautéed in a tablespoon of olive or canola oil.)

millet

1 cup of brown rice, or any whole grains other than wheat, with steamed asparagus and/or broccoli

1 cup of brown rice, or any whole grains other than wheat, with steamed shredded cabbage and bean sprouts

1 cup of brown rice, or any whole grains other than wheat, with steamed bok choy and carrots

1½ cups of Tao of Wellness cereal*

3–4 ounces of organic skinless chicken breast (or turkey breast or any soy product including but not limited to tofu, tempeh, etc.) with steamed kale and mushrooms

½ cup of brown rice with ½ cup of black beans (or any other beans) and steamed zucchini/cauliflower and 3 ounces firm tofu (or organic skinless chicken breast)

1 baked yam or sweet potato with Swiss chard (or any green leafy vegetable) sautéed in water

---

*Tao of Wellness Cereal

(Dr. Mao's Beautiful Hot Herbal Cereal) contains:

Chinese yam (Shan yao)	Lychee (soapberry)
Schisandra (Wu wei zi)	Pearl barley (Yi yi ren)
Long-grain brown rice	Black sesame seeds (Hei zi ma)
Black beans	Poria (Fu ling)
Adzuki beans (Hong dou)	Goji berry (Gou qi zi)
Mixed beans	Fox nut (Qian shi)
Lotus seed (Lian zi)	Sweet rice (Zian mi)

You can also order this premade cereal through the Tao of Wellness website at www.taoofwellness.com.

You may add a pinch of salt, pepper, and up to a tablespoon of walnut oil (unless already used to sauté the chicken or fish or tofu) to any of the above. At dinner, drink 1 cup of detox tea.

Afternoon Snack
8 ounces of vegetable juice and 8 ounces of vegetable broth
  or
1 apple or ½ cup of berries (strawberries, raspberries, etc.)

After Dinner
1 cup of tea (chamomile or Traditions of Tao Internal Cleanse Tea, which is an herbal formula containing chrysanthemum flower, white mulberry leaf, mint leaf, cassia tora seed, dandelion root, shan zha fruit, cocklebur fruit, and licorice root. It is available through www. taoofwellness.com.)

Probiotic Supplement

You may have heard the term *acidophilus,* which is one of the many "good" bacteria and yeasts known as the probiotics. These are living microorganisms that help balance our intestinal functions. These good bacteria help you break down food and assimilate it as well as control the "bad" bacteria that are also found in your system. When you are healthy, these different bacteria are in balance. But when you are sick or stressed, are taking antibiotics on a long-term basis, or are eating an unhealthy diet, this balance is disrupted. In effect, these situations can strip your intestinal lining of probiotics. This is one of the reasons why I would like you to take a probiotic supplement during the detoxification process. You can find acidophilus in capsule form in most health food stores.

Aloe Vera

Aloe Vera is a detox juice that can either be added to the vegetable broth or juice or taken alone (in a 4-ounce serving). It's a good natural cleanser and a great energy booster. It helps with digestion, reduces acid reflux, and helps to reduce allergies. It also controls inflammations in the body and is good for your joints. It is helpful in treating rheumatism and arthritis.

What's in Your Cupboard?
How Healthy Are the Foods You Eat?

When I was a small boy, my mother was a teacher at the same elementary school I attended. I remember how after school she would plunk me on her bicycle and start toward home. As we rode, we would pass farms where we would stop and buy the ingredients for our evening meal. First we would pick up vegetables from farmers who would pull them up from the muddy field and rinse them off quickly before handing them to us.

Next we would go to the open market where they sold foods straight from the earth and water. What we couldn't fit in our basket, we slung over our shoulders. We would buy fresh fish that was still jumping, shellfish that was still crawling. And we'd buy fruit: not the perfect, stackable apples you see today in the supermarket all covered with wax, but apples with blemishes that were tasty enough for the birds to fight over.

Today it's unrealistic to imagine hopping on a bicycle and buying fresh food every day. Even when we do make it to the market and buy fruits and vegetables, we still have to soak them to remove the pesticides. Yes, there is still fresh food. But it's not like when I was a little boy in Taiwan. Those memories of riding on my mother's bike and picking up fresh food stay with me even now. It was a perfect world for me.

There's really no other way around it: food is best in its natural state. In an ideal world, we'd all eat nothing but whole foods that are just as nature made them. But we do not live in an easy world. We run from one activity to another, trying to balance family and work and all the rest of the elements that make up our complicated lives. It's no wonder we rely on convenience foods and so-called fast foods. What kinds of foods are you really getting when you head down that supermarket aisle? If you are relying heavily on frozen, processed, or canned foods, you might be serving your body foods that not only are lacking in nutrition but are also harmful to your health in the long run. What harms your health harms your fertility. Here are some of the biggest offenders.

Coffee

Coffee is a natural stimulant. The caffeine it contains gives you a lift, helps you stay awake, and increases your concentration level—what could be wrong with that? The answer is plenty if you are trying to get pregnant.

The caffeine in coffee stimulates your nervous system, temporarily increasing your heart rate and raising your blood pressure. There is no problem with moderate occasional use. But if you drink coffee on a daily basis, especially as a substitute for a nutritious breakfast, you can compromise your blood sugar levels and create an energy deficit. When that happens, you run the risk of raising your adrenal gland activities as a way to compensate for this loss. That can spell trouble for your fertility, since chronic overactive adrenal glands, when combined with an overstimulated nervous system, can prohibit the proper function of uterine contractions, the tubal functions of transporting the egg, and finally, implantation itself. In short, it can have a suppressive effect on female hormones.

If you don't drink coffee, don't start now. If you drink more than a cup a day, cut back. And if you are over the age of thirty-five and trying to get pregnant, don't drink coffee at all.

Sugar

If sugar is so bad for you, then why are there so many delicious cookies, pastries, and candies in the world? The answer is simple: they taste good. But sugar also happens to be among the most addictive substances known to humankind. When you eat those cookies (simple sugar) or pastries (refined carbohydrates), your pancreas goes on high alert and starts to produce and release insulin.

Insulin is a hormone secreted by your pancreas that helps stabilize your blood sugar levels by regulating your metabolism. When you indulge yourself with a frequent intake of sweets, your pancreas must work overtime to secrete more insulin to catch up with the added sugar. After a while your body becomes accustomed to the elevated insulin state. When that happens, you become resistant to the effects of a normal amount of insulin. This temporary insulin resistance can decrease proper ovarian function and your fertility potential. Too much sugar can also potentially change the quality of your cervical mucus, making it more acidic and less conducive to retaining and protecting sperm. In men, it can actually reduce sperm motility, making sperm unable to swim well enough to meet the woman's egg.

Refined sugar and processed sugars like corn syrup and fructose are just plain bad for you, particularly when you are trying to get pregnant. A snack bar, for example, might say "no added sugar" on the label. But read further and you may find the words "sweetened with fructose or fruit concentrate." Don't be fooled. White, brown, or in liquid form, sugar is sugar. Avoid it or at least reduce your consumption of it. If you are eating grains, fruits, and vegetables, you are already getting enough sugar in a natural form. You do not need more in a refined form.

Processed Foods

Any foods that contain artificial flavor, artificial color, or artificial preservatives fall in the category of processed foods. Eliminate them from your diet altogether if you can. We know they are not good for your body in the long run; in the short run, they can actually place a chemical burden on it.

Think about what happens when you buy a new pair of shoes. The first time you wear them, they might get a little dusty. After a few more wearings, they start to pick up dirt. If you don't clean your shoes at that point, the dirt and the dust will continue to pile up. Pretty soon, that dirt will start to affect both the material and the look of the shoes. At some point, the dirt will become like tar that you won't be able to remove. It's the same with your body. In health, your body is an efficient machine with the ability to detoxify itself. A small amount of chemicals will probably not create that much of a burden on your body's organs and systems. But if you continue to accumulate them over a long period of time, these chemicals can potentially become endotoxic. In effect, they can poison your endocrine and other internal systems and decrease your body's ability to cleanse itself. They can start to interfere with your metabolism and with the conversion of hormones.

So look at your supply of processed, frozen, and prepared foods. Get rid of that box of orange mac-and-cheese, those sodium- and chemical-laden soups, those dinners with artificial flavoring. Read the labels, and don't be fooled just because something comes from the health food store. If you see chemicals in the ingredients, be wary.

Alcohol

I'll be perfectly blunt: no alcohol. Recent scientific studies have suggested that even moderate drinking can decrease fertility potential in both males and females.

Alcohol is hard on the liver. But that's not the only reason for avoiding it while you are trying to get pregnant. In order to have good fertility, your hormones must work in a balanced fashion. Because the liver has a close relationship with both male and female sex hormones, any burden on the liver can change how it assists in the production of these hormones. Alcohol can affect your ovulation, causing it to become irregular. When consumed by your male partner, alcohol can be directly harmful to the sperm. It can weaken, slow, and damage all of the sperm parameters, including their shape, speed, structure, and liveliness. As if that's not enough, drinking alcohol puts you and your baby at higher risk for a miscarriage, preterm birth, stillbirth, and other serious conditions.

You might use alcohol to relax your body and mind after a day of hard work. While I think it is a good idea to unwind on a daily basis, there are many better alternatives for achieving this. Taking a hot bath is one—just make sure it's no more than fifteen minutes at a time. A walk after dinner, drinking noncaffeinated tea, and meditation are also good ways to put yourself at ease.

Monosodium Glutamate

Monosodium glutamate (MSG) is a unique food enhancer that is added to many of the foods we eat. Contrary to popular thinking, it is not just used in Japanese and Chinese restaurants. It can be found in many nonethnic restaurant dishes as well as in canned soup, potato chips, snack foods, and frozen dinners, just to name a few. While most people tolerate a small amount of MSG well, others can be extremely sensitive to it. Symptoms can include burning, numbness, tingling, flushing, or weakness in the face, neck, upper back, forearms, and chest, as well as rapid heartbeat, headache, nausea, and even difficulty breathing. We do know that infants are more sensitive to MSG because their nervous system is weaker and therefore more prone to overstimulation. Make a practice of reading food labels so that you can reduce your intake of MSG.

Dairy

It's true that dairy products are high in protein and calcium. But they are also high in fat. When women who are trying to get pregnant need to gain weight and increase their body fat, I recommend that they actually eat more dairy products. It is the quickest way I know to gain the protein and fat that are necessary for reproductive function. But if your weight is normal, or especially, if you are overweight or obese, keep dairy products to a minimum. If you feel you must eat dairy, go for low or non-fat products. Avoid dairy altogether if you have dairy intolerance marked by bloating, gas, or sinus congestion after consuming dairy products. Intestinal disturbance and allergies can and will interrupt proper endocrine function. Improper endocrine function can in turn cause a thickening of your cervical mucus, resulting in decreased sperm transportation, fertilization, and embryo implantation.

Calcium is an essential nutrient that your body needs to have strong bones, heart, muscles, and nerve functions. It's important for follicular production and general reproductive functions in both men and women. While the best source of calcium is dairy products, there are alternatives such as orange juice or soy milk fortified with calcium, tofu made from calcium sulfate, dark green leafy vegetables, beans, and sardines.

The one dairy product that I absolutely recommend avoiding is butter. It is not a good source of fat. It can wreak havoc on your fertility by clogging up your arteries and decreasing your circulation.

Soda

Soda contains sugar, preservatives, and other synthetic chemicals. Too much soda prohibits you from eating proper nutritive foods that might be good for your health and your fertility potential.

Tap Water

I can hear you now. "No coffee, no sugar, no crunchy snack foods, no wine, no soda . . . and now, no water?" I am simply asking that you drink filtered or bottled water when you are trying to increase your fertility. Unfiltered tap water can contain chemicals. Scientists have told us that tap water is most likely safe to drink, but not all tap water is the same. While occasional consumption of plain tap water is not a problem in developed countries, filtered water is much better for your health in the long run.

Many women ask me how many glasses of water they should drink per day. Some studies recommend as many as eight glasses. I recommend moderation—no more than five glasses or so a day, since you should ideally be getting liquid from food sources like fruits and soup. If you drink too much water, you run the risk of excessive water syndrome, which could cause vital nutrients and trace minerals to be leached from your system.

Make sure the water you drink is not icy cold. As cold water goes down into your stomach, your body warms it up by using energy and circulation that could be put to better use in your pelvic area, your uterus, and your ovaries.

What's in Your Medicine Cabinet?

In Chinese medicine, we believe that drugs should be used only when our natural system cannot manage or do well in healing itself. I believe this with all my heart. When I finished college, my father presented me with a choice: go into Western medicine or Chinese medicine. I was to

---

Women's Voices

"I was optimistic that Chinese medicine would make a huge difference. So I did all the things I was told: no sugar, no caffeine, no frozen bottles of water.... It was the end of the whole journey for me. I wanted to have peace that I did everything I could do before giving up the hope of getting pregnant."

---

do whatever I desired. At that point, I had already had a lot of background in healing and in Taoist principles. As you now know, Taoist principles are all about being in touch with nature. If we can understand nature, then we can draw on its resources to help us heal and strengthen, all with less pain and suffering.

I started to realize that I did not like to use drugs whenever I could find a natural remedy for the condition that I was treating. I already had a strong opinion that we should allow our bodies to heal naturally, instead of controlling the process all the time. To me, drugs were, and still are, like a strong and ruthless army that takes over your body. When I thought about Western medicine, I thought about the time I would have to spend learning about drugs I would not like to use much. This was a philosophical problem—one that involved my personal principles.

I chose Chinese medicine.

Here in the West and in the world in general, we have increasingly become a drug-controlled society. Drugs are chemicals with powerful effects and side effects on the body. Using drugs to solve problems over the long term can create all kinds of imbalances with your internal organs. One drug can create other problems that then require treatment with more drugs. Pretty soon, you are taking several different drugs. You think you might know the interactions, but the truth is that your body slowly becomes more dependent on these drugs and starts to lose its natural functions. And then, of course, there are the side effects. Have you ever listened to commercials for drugs on the radio or television? The announcers barely have time to mention all the possible side effects that can come with taking one particular drug. Take more than one drug, and just imagine the possibilities for side effects and interactions.

If you look in your medicine cabinet, what do you see? Do you see pain relievers, sleeping tablets, pills for headaches or stomachaches or cramps? I am not judging you. But if you need to take these medications on a regular basis, then something is indeed wrong. Masking the pain won't help you understand what is causing it. You need to figure out why your body is calling out for help before you can start to heal it. If you don't and you continue to use drugs simply to ease your symptoms, you might end up with a bigger problem than you bargained for.

A good example is the widespread use of oral contraceptives to help regulate menstrual irregularities. Unquestionably, oral contraceptives have incredible benefits when used as a method of birth control. They forever changed the status of women in this society by allowing them the freedom to choose when—and when not—to get pregnant. It is their secondary use that sometimes causes potential problems.

Let's say you are a young woman who is experiencing pain with your periods. In Western medicine, it's likely your doctor will prescribe oral contraceptives as a remedy. The pill will probably work well to block your pain and regulate your cycles. But if you continue to use it for pain therapy rather than for the purpose of contraception, you might never get to the root of your real problem.

For example, you might be suffering from endometriosis or other conditions that need further investigation. (It should be noted that the only way to definitively diagnose endometriosis is via laparoscopic surgery. There are, however, signs—including painful menstruation and pelvic conditions, and little cysts called endometriomas seen through ultrasounds—that point to endometriosis. If you experience any of these symptoms, it is important to see a doctor for more testing.) But many women put off seeing a doctor because once they start taking the pill, their pain subsides. Perhaps you are even one of them, which means you go along with life only to find out later, when you finally go off the contraceptives to try and get pregnant, that you cannot. What's more, your painful symptoms have likely returned. Whatever problem you masked is still there, and you are now that much older and having trouble getting pregnant. The original problem has been compounded by another. Am I saying that the use of oral contraceptives to deal with pain is a terrible thing? Not at all. If your pain is truly unbearable, even after trying other natural remedies, then it might be the answer. Just know that your fertility potential might be more compromised than other women's when you get older. This knowledge may also help you to make a wiser choice in choosing when to start a family.

In China, girls are taught by their mothers to look at pain in a different way. Pain during your period is a sign that something is not right and that your endocrine system is not in balance. This means you must address it in ways other than with painkillers or birth-control pills. When I was taking care of women in outpatient clinics in China, I saw young girls having great pain with their periods. But their parents would not let them simply take painkillers. Instead, the parents took their daughters for treatments that involved herbs, acupuncture, and lessons in changing their lifestyle and nutritional habits.

The idea of the quick fix versus gradual change is one of the biggest differences between Western and Chinese medicine. I believe your body is smart and is always trying to tell you things. Ultimately, the long-term use of drugs is not good for you, not just because they are strong chemical agents, but because drugs take control and leave your body a passive bystander. They do not allow you to go to the root of the problem. They promote a false sense that everything is fine. This quick fix has a lot of hidden baggage.

People talk a lot about procedures nowadays. Face-lifts, liposuction, and yes, even IVF procedures . . . they sound so easy. Do you carry too much fat? Do you have little patience? Then go for the quick fix. But what most doctors won't tell you is that these quick fixes, these so-called procedures, are surgeries, plain and simple. We treat these procedures as normal, like having breakfast in the morning. But they involve anesthesia, which is very hard on the body and potentially dangerous. General anesthesia can weaken your heart as well as your endocrine system. Often, recovery is slow, which can greatly reduce your health status. That's why you should always explore other alternatives before considering surgery. This is especially important when you are dealing with infertility challenges, as I will discuss later in this book.

There are times where we overdo procedures, especially in the area of imaging. The use of X-ray, MRI, and CT scans has become common in the process of diagnosis. But imaging should be as minimal as possible, since your fertility can be adversely affected by radiation. In preserving your fertility potential, you need to use drugs, surgeries, and radiological procedures conservatively and minimally.

And since we opened your medicine cabinet, there's one more caution I must add. Sometimes what can make you beautiful can also make you sick. I'm speaking about the chemicals found in those cosmetics, shampoos, and creams that line your shelves. Some of them contain trace heavy metals, which can get into your system. Others may contain endocrine-disrupting chemicals that can affect egg quality and sperm quality—or both. Read the labels. You should avoid cosmetics with the following ingredients: imidazolidinyl urea, diazolidinyl urea, methyl paraben, propyl paraben, butyl paraben, ethyl paraben, petrolatum, propylene glycol, PVP/VA copolymer, stearalkonium chloride, synthetic colors, synthetic fragrances, diethanolamine (DEA), monoethanolamine (MEA), triethanolamine (TEA), dioxane, 2-bromo-2-nitropropane-1,3-diol (bronopol), benzalkonium chloride, butylated hydroxyanisole (BHA), butylated hydroxytoluene (BHT), chloromethylisothiazolinone, and isothiazolinone.

Beauty shouldn't come at the price of your health.

Replacing Old Habits with New Ones: A Practical Shopping Guide

Okay, we've thrown out the bad stuff in your pantry and refrigerator. If you still find you have plenty to eat, congratulations! But if you're looking at empty shelves and those never-used vegetable bins, don't despair. Now is the perfect time to replenish your food supply and your health. But first, a few basics.

Why Organic?

Look at the strawberries next time you're in the supermarket. If the store carries both conventionally grown and organic fruits, chances are you can spot the organic strawberries with one glance. In plain words, they are not as pretty as their pesticide-grown sisters. They tend to be smaller and less uniform in color and shape, not to mention more expensive. Then why buy them?

For regular strawberries to grow to such beautiful size with no blemishes, a lot of chemical fertilizers and pesticides have been used. Remember that chemical burden? The more unhealthy chemicals you have in your body, the more energy your body has to expend to detox just so that it can continue its normal functioning. When these chemicals stay in your body, they become disrupters that can potentially decrease and diminish your endocrine function. They can change your cycle, they can change how you ovulate, and they can decrease fertility.

These chemical burdens can also create infertility problems in men. A few recent studies have shown that sperm level has been decreasing worldwide. One hypothesis suggests it's because we're ingesting more and more hormones and other chemicals in food: from the meat and poultry we eat, to milk and cheese, and so on down the food chain.

If you don't have access to organic fruits and vegetables or hormone-free foods, it's not the end of the world (or your fertility!). But it's not a bad idea to be aware of which fruits and vegetables are the highest—and the lowest—in pesticides while buying conventionally grown food. One good source of information is the Environmental Working Group (EWG), a nonprofit organization specializing in environmental investigations. Their website address is www.ewg.org.

What about fish, poultry, and meat? Do you really need to buy only those labeled hormone-free or antibiotic-free? Again, if you have neither the means nor the money to buy solely organic food, it's worthwhile to educate yourself on how much of a risk you are taking by eating certain foods. While there are no advisories for meat and poultry, I would say don't sacrifice nutrition and a balanced diet out of fear. Lean meat and poultry are still wonderful sources of protein. So is fish, although here the benefits and risks are a lot clearer.

For instance, nearly all fish and shellfish contain traces of mercury. For most people, the risk from mercury when eating fish and shellfish is not a health concern. Yet some fish and shellfish contain higher levels of mercury that may harm an unborn baby or young child's developing nervous system. The risks from mercury in fish and shellfish depend on the amount eaten and the levels of mercury they contain. Therefore, the U.S. Food and Drug Administration (FDA) and the Environmental Protection Agency (EPA) are advising women who may become pregnant, pregnant women, nursing mothers, and young children to avoid some types of fish and to eat fish and shellfish that are lower in mercury.

How do you know which fish is safe to eat? For the greatest peace of mind, follow these two basic guidelines:

1. Do not eat shark, swordfish, king mackerel, or tilefish because they contain higher levels of mercury. Be aware that albacore ("white") tuna has more mercury than canned light tuna. Therefore, try and limit your consumption of albacore tuna to one meal (6 ounces) per week.

2. Check local advisories about the safety of fish caught by family and friends in your local lakes, rivers, and coastal areas. If no advice is available, eat up to 6 ounces (one average meal) per week of fish you catch from local waters, but don't consume any other fish during that week. (*Note:* For more information, check the website www.epa.gov/waterscience/fish.)

Balancing the Five Food Groups

Have I scared you enough with warnings about nonorganic foods, processed foods, and mercury-laden fish? Take heart: there are still plenty of wonderful, fertility-enriching, healthy food choices left. A healthy eating plan begins with consuming a wide variety of foods. Favoring or indulging in only one type of food can cause malnourishment and imbalance—a detriment to fertility.

These food groups are a good starting point for you in terms of finding a balanced diet. If you would like more information, the United States Department of Agriculture (USDA) has a useful resource called the Food Guide Pyramid. You can access it on the web at www.mypyramid.gov.

The Vegetable Group

Everyone needs to eat more vegetables and fruits! Many research studies have shown vegetables and fruits to be critical in promoting good health. In fact, they should be the foundation of a healthy diet. Vegetables consist mostly of water and fiber. They are excellent sources of essential vitamins, minerals, and fibers. They also strengthen the body with their disease-fighting phytonutrients. Many aspects of the reproductive system require these nutrients. A healthy diet for fertility should consist of seven to nine servings of vegetables and fruits daily. One serving of fruits and vegetables should fit within the palm of your hand—it's a lot smaller than most people think!

Dark Green Vegetables

Beet greens	Dark green leafy lettuce
Bok choy	Endive
Broccoli	Escarole
Carrot tops	Kale
Chard	Mesclun
Chicory	Mustard greens
Chrysanthemum	Romaine lettuce
greens	Spinach
Collard greens	Turnip greens
Dandelion greens	Watercress

Orange Vegetables

Acorn squash	Pumpkin
Butternut squash	Sweet potatoes
Carrots	Winter squash
Hubbard squash	

Other Vegetables

Artichokes	Bean sprouts
Asparagus	Beets

Breadfruit

Brussels sprouts

Cabbage

Cauliflower

Celery

Chinese cabbage

Corn

Cucumbers

Daikon radish (Japanese white radish)

Eggplant

Green beans

Green or red peppers

Green peas

Hominy

Iceberg (head) lettuce

Mushrooms

Okra

Onions

Radishes

Parsnips

Potatoes

Shiitake mushrooms

Snow peas

Summer squash

Tomato juice

Tomatoes (considered a vegetable in Asia)

Turnips

Vegetable juice

Wax beans

Zucchini

The Fruit Group

Fruits are energy foods. They contain water and sugar, but they also provide you with many essential vitamins, minerals, fiber, and phytonutrients—just like vegetables. Serving size is indicated in parentheses. Where it's not, 1 cup of sliced or cut-up fruit is a good gauge. The majority of commercially prepared fruit juices do not have the same nutrient value as fruits. Most of the valuable fibers have been removed. But juicing a whole fruit is fine if you do not throw away the fiber. Add some pulp to the juice.

Apple (1)

Apricot, dried (3)

Apricot, fresh (2)

Avocado (1)

Banana (1)

Blueberries

Cantaloupe

Carambola (star fruit) (1)

Cherimoya (1)

Cherries (4)

Durian (½)

Figs (2)

Grapefruit (½)

Grapes (1 handful)

Honeydew melon (¼)

Juices, all (¾ cup)

Kiwi (1)

Logan (3)

Loquat (3)

Pineapple

Lychee, fresh or canned (3)

Plum (1)

Mango (1)

Pomegranate (½)

Nectarine (1)

Prunes, dried (4)

Orange (1)

Rambutan (3)

Papaya (½)

Strawberries (4)

Peach (1)

Tangerine (1)

Pear (1)

Watermelon

The Bean Group

Beans are a wonderful source of nutrition. They are high in fiber, low in fat, and a good source of protein. Beans are also rich in folate, iron, and many other vitamins and minerals. This group of foods is essential in developing good follicle quality. Beans also stabilize blood sugar and can be very helpful to people who might be prone to hypoglycemia or insulin resistance.

Adzuki beans

Mung beans

Black beans

Navy beans

Black-eyed peas

Pinto beans

Garbanzo beans
    (chickpeas)

Soybeans

Split peas

Kidney beans

Tofu (bean curd made from
    soybeans)

Lentils

Lima beans (mature)

White beans

The Grain Group

Grains are the most important food group. Grains provide complex carbohydrates that supply energy. They are also a rich source of vitamins and minerals. Grains are low in fat, high in fiber, and cholesterol-free. They are at the base of the Food Pyramid because we need more servings from this group of foods than from any other group.

Grains are divided into two subgroups: whole grains and refined grains. Whole grains are more nutritious than refined grains because nutrients have not been lost in processing. Whole grains contain the entire grain kernel—the bran, germ, and endosperm. Refined grains have been milled, a process that removes the bran and germ. This is done to give grains a finer texture and improve their shelf life, but it also removes dietary fiber, iron, and many B vitamins. Most refined grains are enriched; that is, certain B vitamins (thiamine, riboflavin, niacin, folic acid) and iron are added back after processing. Fiber, however, is usually not added back to enriched grains.

While many of our grain food choices are a mixture of whole and refined grains, it's more nutritious to put the emphasis on whole grains, especially brown rice, whole wheat, amaranth, quinoa, barley, and triticale.

Whole Grains—Desirable

Amaranth	Oatmeal
Barley	Rye flakes
Brown rice	Sorghum
Buckwheat	Teff
Buckwheat noodles	Triticale
Bulgur (cracked wheat)	Wheat berries
Corn grits	Whole cornmeal
Granola (grains mixture)	Whole-grain cereals
Millet	(mixed grains)
Muesli (mixed grains)	Whole-wheat flour
Oat bran	Wild rice
Oat groats	

Refined Grains—Not Desirable

Cornflakes	Refined noodles
Degermed cornmeal	Refined spaghetti
Flour tortillas	Refined pitas
Refined corn bread	Refined pretzels
Refined corn tortillas	White bread
Refined couscous	White rice
Refined crackers	White sandwich buns
Refined macaroni	and rolls

The Meat Group

Meat by definition is all animal tissue for food consumption. All flesh is very high in protein, containing all of the essential amino acids. Flesh is usually very low in carbohydrates. Red meat, such as beef, pork, and lamb, contains many essential nutrients such as iron, zinc, and protein necessary for healthy growth and development as well as for general well-being. (Fruits and vegetables, by contrast, usually lack several essential amino acids.)

Fish is rich in polyunsaturated fatty acids called omega-3s: mainly, eicosapentaenoic acid (EPA; in saltwater fish) and docosahexaenoic acid (DHA). These omega-3s reduce the inflammatory process in blood vessels and improve microcirculation. This can be helpful in improving blood flow to the reproductive organs such as the uterus and ovaries. Eating fish can decrease heart disease and therefore has better health benefits than eating red meat.

Land Meat

Beef	Pork
Chicken	Turkey
Lamb	

Water Meat—Fish

Catfish	Pollack
Cod	Salmon
Crab	Shark
Flounder	Shellfish
Hake	Swordfish
Halibut	Tuna

The key is to eat a variety of foods from all of the five groups. (A sixth group, dairy, has not been included, since dairy products are used sparingly in a traditional Chinese medicine food program.) As a general rule of thumb, if you are not overweight, are between twenty and fifty years old, and are moderately active, you should consume about 2,000 to 2,200 calories per day (compared to the 2,400 to 2,800 calories per day recommended for men). The most important message I can give you is to concentrate on simple food, and make sure you don't skip meals. Nourishment is essential to your fertility.

THE POWER OF HERBS

*The natural essence of the universe
gives life to all things.*

—FROM *THE COMPLETE WORKS OF LAO TZU*
TRANSLATION AND ELUCIDATION BY HUA-CHING NI

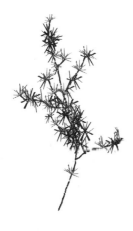

One summer during my childhood, I had a very bad toothache that began around noontime. By two o'clock, my toothache was so severe that I was begging for an acupuncture treatment to ease the pain. My mother, wise woman that she was, told me that I had too much "fire" and proceeded to go into our garden to get some herbs. I watched as she washed and blended the herbs into a thick juice. Then she handed it to me to drink.

I can still remember how miserably bitter the taste was. Of course, I protested. My mother calmly responded that the bitter taste was good for quenching the fire and that I must drink the whole cup. I did, reluctantly, then fell asleep almost immediately afterward. When I woke up two hours later, not only was my toothache gone, but in its place I felt a sense of coolness and well-being throughout my whole body. I felt so well that I was able to resume my noisy and annoying teenage behavior immediately. Later, I found out that the herb was dandelion, a cooling herb frequently used for fire conditions such as toothaches, headaches, and nosebleeds.

There were many other similar incidents like this one throughout my childhood. I didn't fully understand the power of herbs until I was old enough to work in the herb room. I was thirteen at the time. Under my father's instruction, I was taught to memorize each herb's functions and how it could serve the body. I remember having to learn ten different herbs each day. I did this for three months every summer. If I could recite the functions of these ten herbs back to my father, then I could go out and play.

There are over a thousand common herbal formulas—more, if you include the traditional family formulas developed over generations. Fortunately, my father set a reasonable goal for me in my childhood, leaving plenty of time to play.

When I prescribe an herbal treatment, I'm often asked how I arrive at the proper formula. Like everything else in Chinese medicine, your herbal treatment would be based on your constitution, your environment, and your medical condition and needs. And a lot of it is trial and error.

A typical formula is made from about ten to fifteen herbs. I like to call this practice a synergistic approach. Herbs are combined not only to maximize their effects but so that the formula can be used to address a wider variety of problems. If one herb doesn't do the trick, another will. The skill is in knowing the properties of each herb and how they all work together. By combining different herbs in different quantities, you end up with the desired result. As a patient's needs and condition change, so will the formula. Sometimes it's necessary to change it on a weekly basis.

Women's Voices

"I drank the teas. I never found them revolting, but I wouldn't choose it in a restaurant! But they became part of my life. Even though I have my child now, I still take them to feel healthy."

Dr. Dao's Ten Favorite Fertility Herbs

NUMBER	COMMON NAME	PIN YIN NAME	PHARMACEUTICAL NAME	BOTANICAL NAME
1	Dodder seeds	Tu si zi	Semen Cuscutae	Cuscuta chinensis
2	Chinese goji berry, or Chinese wolfberry	Gou qi zi	Fructus Lycii	Lycium barbarum
3	Morinda root	Ba ji tian	Radix Morindae Officinalis	Morinda officinalis
4	Cistanches	Rou cong rong	Herba Cistanches	Cistanche salsa
5	Epimedium	Xian ling pi	Herba Epimedii	Epimedium grandiflorum
6	Milk-vetch root	Huang qi	Radix Astragali	Astragalus membranaceus
7	Chinese angelica root	Dang qui	Radicis Angelicae Sinensis	Angelica sinensis
8	Chinese foxglove root	Shu di huang	Radix Rehmanniae Preparata	Rehmannia glutinosa
9	Asiatic cornelian cherry	Shan zhu yu	Fructus Corni	Cornus officinalis
10	Chinese yam	Shan yao	Rhizoma Dioscoreae	Dioscorea opposita

Still, certain herbs have stood the test of time when it comes to fertility and Chinese medicine. I have provided you with my top ten. If you look at the table, you will see it is divided into sections. Common Name refers to the name of the herb as it might be called in a health food store. Pin Yin refers to the system of romanization for standard Mandarin. Romanization basically means using Roman letters to represent sounds in Mandarin rendering. The Pharmaceutical Name column shows the name you might see in Whole Foods or other health food stores. It refers to the part of the plant that has been used for the medicine. The Botanical Name is the name of the plant, along with its family and species.

1. Dodder Seeds

Dodder seeds are derived from two similar species of plants: *Cuscuta chinensis Lam* and *Cuscuta japonica Choisy.* It is a powerful herb that has multitudes of therapeutic benefits for both men and women. In men, it can improve many different aspects of semen production as well as reduce abnormal sperm chromosomal issues. In women, I like to use it to strengthen egg quality and to induce better ovulation. It is also good in thickening the uterine lining and helpful in cases where a woman has an elevated FSH (follicle-stimulating hormone) level, or is a poor responder to IVF or IUI (intrauterine insemination).

2. Chinese Goji Berry

Known for its antiaging characteristics, these sweet-tasting berries are high in antioxidants and vitamins C, B1, and B2. They are very effective in treating infertility issues in both men and women. In women, goji berry stimulates the uterus to thicken the lining, which is important for fetus implantation. It is also helpful in strengthening follicular quality. In men, Chinese clinical studies found it to be effective in improving both motility and sperm count within one to two months.

3. Morinda Root

This herb is particularly effective in treating female infertility. A mild thyroid fortifier, it also improves thyroid function. Morinda root treats symptoms that often accompany menstruation. These include cold and painful limbs, dull lower abdominal pain, and pain and coldness in the lower back region. It stimulates the blood circulation around the uterus and increases implantation rate.

Morinda root is also traditionally used to strengthen the muscles and tendons. Besides providing better blood flow to the uterus, it treats musculoskeletal aches and pains during pregnancy and may decrease the risk of miscarriage.

Morinda root is effectively used in treating male infertility accompanied by signs of sexual weakness such as premature ejaculation and low libido.

4. Cistanche

This plant is one of my favorite herbs because of its effectiveness in treating infertility while also helping to regulate the bowels and cleanse the body of unnecessary waste. In men, we use cistanche to help restore the necessary sexual fire and vitality to the body. We use it in women to warm the uterus, thereby improving blood circulation and hormonal release in that particular area. It is beneficial during the proliferation phase of a woman's cycle, as it supports the release and effectiveness of progesterone. With this increased hormonal function and circulatory effect, cistanche indirectly promotes the thickening of a woman's uterine lining, thus providing a greater chance for implantation. It also assists with the effects stemming from the loss of blood and nourishment during a woman's period.

5. Epimedium

This herb has a long history of use in fertility and sexual dysfunction. It increases sperm production in men, and stimulates desire for sexual activity in both men and women—known in Chinese medicine as "stoking the fire within." It has been shown to increase production of hormones such as corticosterone, cortisol, and testosterone. Epimedium has also been shown to have pharmacological functions similar to testosterone, which helps women and men in strengthening libido.

In laboratory tests, epimedium has been shown to reduce blood pressure by dilating the arteries, especially the coronary arteries. It helps increase oxygen circulation and reduce cholesterol while strengthening immune function.

6. Milk-Vetch Root

Milk-vetch root has been commonly used as supportive treatment for anemia, chronic fatigue, and cancer. It is known widely for its immune-modulating and immune-boosting functions. Patients with frequent colds and other illnesses tend to have weak constitutions, in which case this herb is especially helpful. Combining it with Chinese angelica root creates a powerful duet commonly used in all types of anemia and chronic fatigue conditions. In reproductive medicine, milk-vetch root is very useful in situations of anemia, hypothyroidism, poor uterine lining development, and postpartum recovery. It is also widely used to enhance the body's insulin sensitivity and is currently under investigation in treating insulin resistance in patients with polycystic ovarian syndrome.

I frequently use this herb as a principal herb, combining it with many other herbs in a formula to address the needs of patients with multiple challenges of infertility (especially age-related, uterine, and ovulatory factors).

7. Chinese Angelica Root

This blood-enriching herb has been used in China for over a thousand years to help regulate women's menstrual cycles. Its Chinese name—*dang gui*—literally means "should return," a reference to its ability to stimulate a woman's period or bring it back to a regular cycle. It does this by nourishing and strengthening the hormonal component of blood as it supports the ovaries' production of estrogen. By increasing blood circulation to the uterus before and during a woman's period, angelica root promotes the completion of the shedding of the endometrial lining. This reduces pain caused by stagnation and incomplete shedding. In addition, angelica root has been an important herb for women with infertility approaching menopause because it nourishes the hormonal component of the blood, providing many of the necessary raw materials for the production of estrogen. It has been used in combination with other herbs to treat anemia, insomnia, and other sleep disorders.

8. Chinese Foxglove Root

Chinese foxglove root is probably the most important herb in Chinese medicine for supporting a woman's menstrual cycle and for nourishing the different hormonal aspects of the blood. I am constantly including both this root and Chinese angelica root in formulas because they work so well together to support the ovaries and hormone production as well as follicular development and the all-important thickening of the uterine lining. Chinese foxglove root helps increase red blood cell production and is used when there are signs of anemia and a decreased menstrual flow. Because it is so effective in nourishing and replenishing the blood and the body's reserves, it is often described as an antiaging herb.

9. Asiatic Cornelian Cherry

Asiatic cornelian cherry is a small, sour cherry from the cornel dogwood tree. It has a wonderful sour taste with an astringent effect in cases of excessive urination and uterine bleeding. It is used in infertility as a nourishing herb to support the hormonal component of the blood. The astringent quality holds the period to full term and supports the function of the fertilized egg holding onto the uterus, thereby reducing instances of miscarriage. It is also used to address insomnia due to hormonal deficiencies.

10. Chinese Yam

This herb is one of my favorite herbs for cooking. It is especially good in soups and bean dishes. Chinese yam assists the pancreatic function of breaking down foods and nutrients within the digestive tract. It also helps the body regulate blood sugar levels. In fact, it has been effectively used in the treatment of diabetes for hundreds of years in China. Modern research has confirmed the Chinese yam's effect in modulating blood glucose fluctuations. It is ideal for those with blood sugar sensitivity and prediabetic symptoms. Chinese yam strengthens and enhances endocrine function. It is ideal for women suffering from infertility because it is a milder-acting herb than many of the others and can be easily introduced into your diet.

What You Can Do on Your Own

Obviously, you are not going to run out and find these herbs and make your own formula—that's a job for a Chinese medical practioner. But if you weren't my patient or couldn't see a Chinese medical practitioner, there are certain over-the-counter herbs and supplements that could be very helpful in improving your fertility. Before getting into specifics, it helps to have an understanding of the difference between herbs and supplements.

Herbs are mostly botanicals, which means they are basically whole forms of some kind of plant. An herb could be part of the plant; it could be the roots, the seeds, the leaves, the fruit—they all have some therapeutic value. Supplements are normally extracts of a natural food source. For example, vitamin A can be extracted from carrots; vitamin C can be extracted from rose hips. So herbs and supplements are a little different, yet they both have similar purposes and similar effects: mainly, to nourish your body and strengthen your body's function. Is one better than the other? Not necessarily. The key is to use them in appropriate ways.

The first supplement I would suggest is a multivitamin with prenatal features—we call them *prenatal vitamins.* The difference between prenatal vitamins and multiple vitamins is that prenatal vitamins have more iron and folic acid and other ingredients to help you get pregnant and to keep your baby healthy once you are. Second, I would recommend that you take some kind of *fish oil,* which is not only very helpful in balancing your fat and cholesterol but can also reduce inflammation in your body. Less inflammation, especially in the pelvic area, could help you get pregnant much more easily. Fish oil improves blood flow, which can help with uterine lining development. I would suggest fish oil that is USP (United States Pharmacy) certified. That requires the manufacturer to adhere to more stringent standards that reduce the amount of mercury and pesticides contained in the product.

Third, I would suggest *L-carnitine* and *L-arginine.* L-carnitine is a derivative of the amino acid lysine. It is essential in energy metabolism and slows down the aging process. L-arginine, another amino acid, is important in helping the endocrine system function in the optimal state. A combination of both can help enhance egg quality and blood flow for uterine lining development. They should be taken during the period when you are trying to conceive. You can discontinue use once you become pregnant.

These are your basic supplements, all of which should be readily available in your local health food store. They are not Chinese herbs. Because herbs are usually stronger than supplements, taking them requires a little more professional guidance and advice. But there are some herbs that you can buy over the counter at most health food stores that are beneficial to fertility and, more important, safe to take long term.

In Chinese medicine, herbs are not just botanicals but are defined as any natural substances or materials that have therapeutic value. The biggest group consists of the botanicals, but minerals and animal products are also a part of the herb world in Chinese medicine. *Royal jelly* is one example. Basically, royal jelly is the honey from the queen bee, which makes it an animal product. It is high in nutrients and contains a tremendous amount of nourishment. We frequently use it for disease recovery in people who are not allergic to honey. We also use it in people who are weakened by anemia. If you are tired, have weak energy, or your life is stressful, this herb is a good one to consider.

Maca root, a Peruvian herb grown at high altitudes, is much like ginseng in its energy-boosting properties. It is a strong antioxidant that is rich in antiaging properties and is generally good for your vitality. It is also very good for reducing sugar cravings, balancing blood sugar, and strengthening circulation. In short, maca root is beneficial for overall reproductive health. My only caution is that this herb comes in different formulas. Make sure the one you take does not contain caffeine.

I've already talked about *goji berry's* amazing qualities when describing my top ten fertility herbs. This truly is a miracle herb. If I were to make an antiaging elixir for women over thirty-five, I would include it. When you combine it with other herbs, it works synergistically and becomes stronger.

You can take goji berries alone. The herb comes in different forms. You can buy dried goji berries and make them into a tea by steeping them. Afterward, you can eat the berries. There are also concentrates that you put into water. Goji berries are very good for blood sugar metabolism and are widely used to treat hypoglycemia. If you get hungry easily and must eat or you will become irritable, this is an extremely helpful herb. In effect, it helps to balance the blood. It is also very good for your eyes. It helps nearsightedness and all kinds of degenerative eye problems. But for women trying to improve their fertility, its greatest gift is strengthening egg quality.

The *raspberry* is very good for improving egg quality. It is a food-grade herb. When taken in food form, it stabilizes blood sugar, strengthens your eyes, and most importantly in terms of your fertility, strengthens your uterine lining. It also relaxes the uterus, which can help to prevent miscarriages. These beneficial properties explain why the raspberry has come to be commonly and safely used during pregnancy, childbirth, and breast-feeding. It's rich in iron, calcium, manganese, and magnesium. And as an added bonus, it can give you beautiful skin.

Aside from the raspberry fruit itself, there are *raspberry leaves*. We don't use the leaves clinically as much in Chinese medicine. But they have similar properties to the berry: they contain vitamins B1, B3, and E, which are all valuable in the promotion of a healthy pregnancy. Raspberry leaves are known to improve fertility, breast milk production, and menstrual regularity. The leaves regulate blood flow, which can be very important when you have irregular periods. Controlling blood flow is also key during labor. In addition, raspberry leaves are used in the treatment of diarrhea, sore throat, and fever.

Vitex is not a Chinese herb but an American one. It is also known as *chaste tree berry*. It is used to regulate periods and to control excessive menstrual flow. It is helpful in treating people who have high levels of male hormones or high levels of prolactin, which is a hormone produced and secreted by the anterior pituitary gland, located in the midbrain area. Prolactin stimulates the mammary glands to produce milk. Too much prolactin, however, can disrupt ovulation and your menstrual cycle.

And then there are herbs that help to promote restful sleep. Getting enough sleep is one of the most important things you can do to help improve your fertility. One that I recommend is *valerian,* a root that comes in both capsule and tea form. It contains properties that help soothe you so that you can get the rest you need. Another herb worth investigating is *schizandra,* which is usually found in berry form. Finally, there's *melatonin,* which is actually a supplement, not an herb. It's a natural substance that is secreted by your body to help regulate your circadian clock, the internal mechanism that determines your sleep cycle. You should stop using melatonin once you become pregnant and while breast-feeding.

ACUPUNCTURE—
RESTORING HARMONY

The subtle Way of the universe
Appears to lack strength,
Yet its power is inexhaustible.

FROM *THE COMPLETE WORKS OF LAO TZU,*
TRANSLATION AND ELUCIDATION BY HUA-CHING NI

The best way to think of acupuncture is as a reset button for your system. Unlike drugs, it is not interventional. It doesn't take over your body. It does help restore balance.

Women's Voices

"There was an immediate and dramatic effect in my body from the first treatment. It's gratifying, and I could feel the difference. Before inserting the needles, Dr. Dao explained I could have one of two reactions. I could react in a neutral way, where I wouldn't see anything at all—or I could be someone overly affected by the treatment. And I was. I saw colors, lights, everything."

Acupuncture, like everything else in Chinese medicine, is based on the observation of our natural environment. Our body is like a little universe. If we stimulate certain areas—what we call points, energy areas, or energy centers—we can also stimulate the inside of our body. This stimulation, in effect, can cause certain physiological changes in blood flow, nerve impulses, healing, and immunological responses, to name a few.

When we insert very fine, stainless steel, surgical-grade, disposable, sterilized needles at these points, your body naturally reacts. Imagine what it would say if it could talk to you: "Hey! I'm here—listen to me. Your arm is injured, or your uterus is weak, or your ovaries are not ovulating well. Your circulation is weak in this whole area, you are not secreting hormones properly, and your body is not reacting or is not

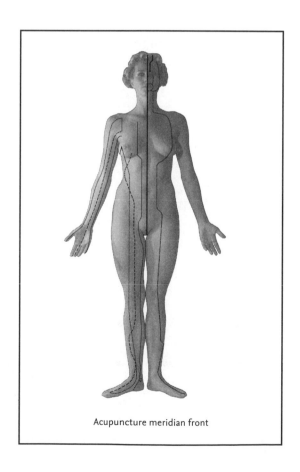

Acupuncture meridian front

sensitive to your hormone secretions. Your egg quality is poor." So much response to little needles!

Of course, knowing where to put the needles is all-important. Where did this knowledge come from? The simple answer is through centuries of trial and error. Countless acupuncture doctors before me figured out that when you stimulate a certain point, you get a certain response that will be good for certain conditions in that area. In fact, you could argue that acupuncture was first used by tribes living thousands of years ago.

Consider this scenario: A poor tribesman is really suffering from back pain. He cannot go out hunting; he cannot go gather fruits. His tribal people think he's worthless and are ready to write him off. So now, besides being in pain, this man is furious. Fed up, he limps off, doubled over, into the wilderness, where he steps smack onto a sharp rock. He starts screaming from the stabbing pain in the bottom of his foot. The tribal elder rushes over and demands to know what is going on. Why does the tribesman have a big rock in his foot? Can't he see that it's stabbing him? And all the while, the tribesman is hopping around, pleading for the elder to help him.

So the elder pulls the sharp rock out and the bleeding eventually stops. The tribesman starts walking in circles, still crying about how much his foot hurts. But the elder is not listening to the complaints; he's too busy noticing something strange. The tribesman is walking! His back is straight!

The tribesman stops in his tracks. The elder is right. His foot is killing him, but his back has never felt better. The tribesman suddenly looks over at the rock. It must be magic! So he picks it up and takes a closer look. Light dawns.

He thinks about his bloody foot and the rock. It went into the right place on his foot. That must be part of the magic. So the tribesman, armed with his rock and his new knowledge, goes around to the others, because he knows that he is not the only one in the tribe with back pain. There are ten more people lying down, ready to be drummed out of the tribe because they can't go out and hunt animals and do other things they need to do to survive. The tribesman takes the sharp rock and stabs each of his fellow sufferers in the exact same location on the bottom of their feet. Immediately every one of them starts to protest.

They rise as one to chase him. Then suddenly . . . they realize. Their back pain is gone, too!

They put the rock on an altar and pray before it. And each time someone's back hurts, the elders take the rock and stab the sufferer in the foot.

Am I telling you a story? Yes, but it's probably not far from the truth. In its crudest form, that was the beginning of acupuncture. We are all scientists when you really think about it. We discover things by observing nature. That's why it's not so far-fetched to imagine one of our ancestors feeling better after accidentally stabbing himself with a sharp rock. What's more, that act undoubtedly led to other discoveries.

In the beginning, acupuncture needles were sharp rocks. Then needles were eventually made from bones, then from bronze, iron, steel, and now, from surgical-grade stainless steel.

Going back to the story of the tribesman and the rock: Eventually people realized that the body will heal if given the right conditions and stimulation. From stabbing a single point on the body to stimulate healing, they progressed to trying to massage certain areas of the body. Very slowly, they started to develop a system. They found different body points that proved helpful for certain body problems. They named these points. Then these points were assigned numbers so that foreign doctors could learn them more easily without having to learn Chinese. Today, for example, we know that when we insert a needle in the point Stomach 36, the stomach can immediately feel better. It restores the balance of digestion.

What is the physiological explanation? We do know that acupuncture facilitates the release of endogenous opiates like endorphins. These endorphins stimulate the body's self-regulatory mechanism—the biological chemicals that help our body to heal and rejuvenate. But since these endorphins are also part of the endocrine system, they help to improve serotonin secretion in the brain, a kind of feel-good mood hormone that helps us feel better.

One of the most common acupuncture points is at the very top of the head. It's the place where all the energies of our body converge. Needless to say, it is an extremely powerful point used for many purposes, including fertility.

Women's Voices

"I really liked the sense of calmness. . . . I could feel everything circulating after the needles went in during my treatments. It was like everything was letting go."

Does it hurt when the needles go in? The answer is no. In fact, they trigger a very nice calming feeling throughout the body. That's why that point on the top of your head—*baihui*—is so important. Literally translated, it means "the meeting of the hundreds." If you are tense and stressed, you can be sure it will be included in your treatment, as well as if you are suffering from irregular sleep, depression, or anxiety—all of which are fairly common if you are having trouble conceiving. This one particular point is where the yang energy of your body converges.

What exactly is yang energy? In Chinese medicine, we view the body as a reservoir of energies. Within this reservoir are two types of energy: yin and yang. Imagine the yin-yang symbol of the Tao. So, too, do these energies flow in the body. Yin is the material foundation of the body—the muscles, the bones, the joints, the sinews, the tendons, and the tissues—whatever makes up the body. Yin energy tends to settle. Yang energy is something entirely different. It is the actual function of the body. Yang energy is your beating heart, your breathing, your digestive system, your nervous system. Yang energy tends to rise. By stimulating this place on the top of your head, we are allowing yang energy to converge. In this way, we can strengthen your hormones and your endocrine functions. This point is considered the master point of your endocrine and nervous systems.

Another specific point worth mentioning is *fenchi,* located behind your neck. Known as "the pond of wind," it is a point that frequently carries the physical tension of the body. It is very good for regulating blood pressure and blood circulation and for relieving neck and head pains. Rather than causing pain, those tiny needles can relieve it and contribute to a general sense of peace and well-being.

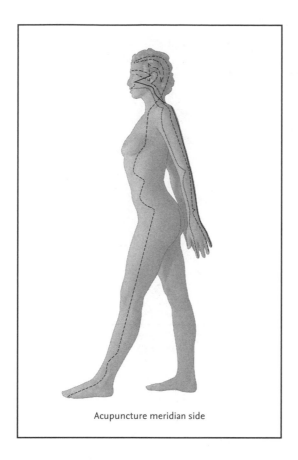

Acupuncture meridian side

We know that if we put a needle in a certain point on the body and then do an imaging study of the brain, we can actually see certain areas of the brain "light up." Obviously, the needles stimulate some part of our nervous system—which only stands to reason, since our body systems are interconnected. The body is really a network of neurons and circulatory channels. There are channels and electrical conduits throughout the body. Therefore, if you stimulate one area, it's going to affect another area. This concept forms the foundation of the holistic perspective underlying Chinese medicine. Distally and proximally, everything is connected within the body, like a network.

As I mentioned, this knowledge didn't come overnight. Trial and error played a great part. Remember our tribesman with the sore back? He finally figured out that he had to stab a particular part of his foot to make

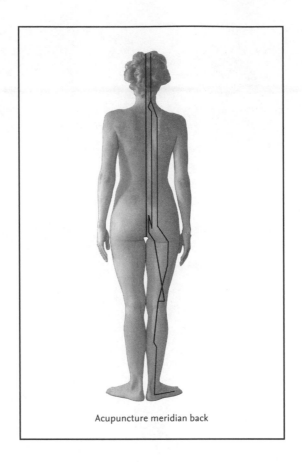

Acupuncture meridian back

his pain go away; that is, he found the correct neural response. Now, suppose he stabbed his foot in the wrong spot one day. His back didn't feel better—but amazingly enough, his neck did. He took note of it and started to consider an idea: What if all the answers to his pain problems could be found in his foot?

That's certainly what foot reflexologists believe. By manipulating and massaging the microsystem of the foot, they treat the entire body system and address all health problems. There's a branch of acupuncture practiced by the Koreans that treats only the hand. In general, though, Chinese acupuncture uses the body acupuncture system. It takes the entire body into consideration—the meridians, the systems, and the points. There are three hundred sixty basic channel points. If you consider all the extra points, the number rises to more than a thousand.

How does acupuncture help in treating infertility? It improves blood flow to the uterus and the reproductive system. This has been shown to help primarily with the implantation of embryos, especially during IVF. It also raises levels of stress-coping hormones such as cortisol and prolactin when it is applied just before ovulation. By decreasing the body's stress response, we increase the chance of fertilization and implantation.

But the number one goal of acupuncture in fertility treatments is the regulation of menstruation and ovulation. That includes beginning and ending your period in a timely and correct manner and making sure your flow is smooth and unhindered, without large clots and without excessive cramps. Acupuncture also helps to strengthen your ovulatory functions and is very good in improving blood flow and building uterine lining quality. And, as previously noted, we have found that acupuncture treatments can be helpful in encouraging implantation of the embryo, which is especially important for women using assisted reproductive techniques. In the last few years, published research studies have shown significant increases in IVF pregnancy rates with the use of acupuncture treatments conjunctively. In fact, I have designed a protocol for the use of acupuncture during IVF that has yielded a significantly better pregnancy rate in a pilot study.

In summary, acupuncture is very good for fertility and for your general health. It resets your circadian clock, reduces stress, helps you release endorphins, and adjusts your endocrine system. It also gets rid of underlying inflammation and solicits immunological balance. Best of all, acupuncture has minimal side effects, and in a skilled hand, is virtually pain-free. (In Chapter 6, we'll learn how to do acupressure, which calls for self-applied pressure rather than needles.)

Our science is still too primitive to fully understand how acupuncture works. In a future century, people will look back at today's science and see that what we know is not that far removed from the early knowledge of the tribesmen. You could say that we are only now just beginning to understand how the human body works.

EXERCISE—THE KEY
TO BALANCE

The subtle essence of the universe is active.
It is like an unfailing fountain of life
Which flows forever in a vast and profound valley.

FROM *THE COMPLETE WORKS OF LAO TZU*,
TRANSLATION AND ELUCIDATION BY HUA-CHING NI

Exercise is very beneficial to your health, especially when you are trying to have a baby. It improves your circulation and helps to get your blood flowing into the various parts of your reproductive system. Why is this so important in terms of your fertility?

Imagine a small body of water. If the water is stagnant, it becomes a swamp that attracts mosquitoes and toxins. Water that doesn't flow becomes stale. But if the water is always flowing, it will always be fresh. Fresh water contains nutrients that help all manner of life to grow—the same way that fresh blood pumping through your system helps provide the nutrients needed for good egg quality. In turn, good egg quality will help with fertilization and implantation, ultimately giving you the chance for a more viable pregnancy. So, first and foremost, exercise is the mechanism that gets your blood flowing.

Exercise boosts your fertility in another way. It increases your endocrine function and stimulates your endocrine glands. These glands are basically organs that secrete the chemical substances we know as hormones. Hormones such as progesterone and estrogen are important to all of us because they help regulate how we grow and develop, among other things. They also play a key role in reproductive functions. They help to make the egg grow, they strengthen egg quality, and they regulate your menstrual cycle. When you exercise regularly and have better circulation, these endocrine functions will become more regular. Exercise also reduces stress—one of the main stumbling blocks on the road to fertility.

The first thing many people think of when they hear the word *exercise* is weight control. But if you are exercising to increase your fertility potential, it is important not to exercise strenuously. I like to break exercise down into three distinct levels: strenuous, moderate, and light.

Running for miles, hiking for hours, doing a triathlon . . . these activities are examples of what I would consider strenuous exercise. They are good for weight control and for reducing body fat. But that doesn't necessarily mean they are good for your fertility. Your body is smart; it knows when you require more energy. As you get older, there is a redirection of energy, with or without exercise. Energy shifts away from your reproductive system to the parts of your body that need it more. If you engage in strenuous exercise, your energy goes straight to your muscles, your skeleton, and your heart. That's a long way from your ovaries, where the same energy could be used to produce better-quality eggs.

There are exceptions, of course. I had a thirty-nine-year-old patient who got pregnant while climbing one of the highest peaks in Peru. But she was accustomed to strenuous exercise. She'd been a triathlete almost all of her life. Thus the definition of strenuous really depends on what your body is used to. If you are accustomed to a high level of physical activity, your body comes to expect it. If you don't have that level, you can actually become depressed because your hormone levels drop. That's why it's necessary to ease down by gradually modifying your level of activity. Instead of running, for example, walk for an hour. In general, though, it's wise to curtail heavy energy-burning activity when you are trying to get pregnant. Body fat does make a difference in fertility: too little and it might hinder your chances of getting pregnant. Once you are no longer trying to conceive or maintain a pregnancy, you can resume almost any exercise you are used to. The important thing is to know your body well. Do what you need to do to stay happy, without depleting all your energy resources.

At the other end of the spectrum, there is mild exercise. These are your basic daily activities: walking from your car to your office, moving from your front door to your driveway to pick up your newspaper, lifting groceries out of your car. If your level of activity falls in this category, I would advise you to do more. It's not enough physical exertion, especially if you want to get your blood flowing and depositing nutrients where they are most needed.

Moderate exercise is the best choice when trying to boost your fertility. Examples are gentle cycling, a well-paced walk, or, if you enjoy the gym, thirty minutes on an elliptical machine. Often I hear women complain that it is just too hard to start exercising, especially when they are preoccupied with the process of trying to have a baby. If you are not used to regular exercise, it is always difficult to start. There are ways that you can entice yourself to get moving. One is to get a support system going. Setting up an appointment to exercise with a friend is frequently helpful. Or join a gym: once you pay for the membership, you'll feel guilty if you don't use it.

Different body types require different levels of exercise. For the purpose of helping your fertility, do not overexercise. My strongest recommendation is a combination of walking and some kind of meditative exercise with a focus on breathing and strengthening individual parts of your body. One of the best exercise methods is chi gong.

Chi gong is a series of traditional Chinese exercises that have been passed down for thousands of years. Used for enhancing health, they are quiet, gentle, meditative movements that incorporate specific breathing and concentration techniques. Chi gong has been known to be very helpful in self-healing. There are chi gong rehabilitation centers throughout China that help people with diseases such as cancer, arthritis, and autoimmune disorders. Whereas doing strenuous exercises can make you feel tired afterward, chi gong leaves you feeling peaceful yet energized. Chi gong directs energy to your body to help nourish it internally. If you have any doubts that it could work, know that the Chinese have been practicing it for more than twenty-five hundred years. Twenty million people can't all be wrong!

Over twenty-plus years in my practice, I have seen many women helped by the chi gong exercises that I teach. Those who diligently practice chi gong have seen their uterine fibroids shrink, their chronic pain leave their body, and their fertility restored. These exercises are all about harnessing your own healing power and energy from nature.

Chi Gong Exercise Program

There are ten meditative poses in this program. They should be practiced in order at least twice a day. After waking and before bedtime are preferable, but these poses can be practiced any time of the day as long as your stomach is not full from eating.

You will need a quiet environment like a bedroom that is well ventilated but not too cold. Make sure it's a place where you can stand and sit comfortably (an upright chair is fine), as well as lie flat (on a comfortable floor or a bed). Try not to interrupt the sequence; complete all ten poses in consecutive order unless one of them causes you discomfort. You can begin by holding and practicing a pose for one minute. Later, when you are more comfortable with the exercises, increase the time to three minutes per pose. (These exercises can be practiced any time of the month, regardless of menstruation.)

Allow your emotions and your mind to quiet as you begin your practice. Breathe more slowly and deeply, and allow your body to relax in all of the poses. Once you have become familiar with them, all of these poses are done with your eyes closed.

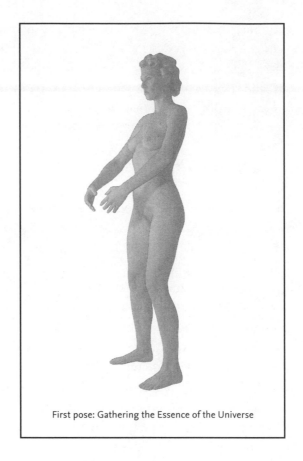

First pose: Gathering the Essence of the Universe

First Pose: Gathering the Essence of the Universe

Stand with your feet shoulder-width apart, knees slightly bent, arms and hands held out in front of you as if you're embracing a small inflated balloon. Your fingers are relaxed and your palms face your pelvic area. Close your eyes and imagine that you are attracting a balloon of heat into this space just in front of your pelvis.

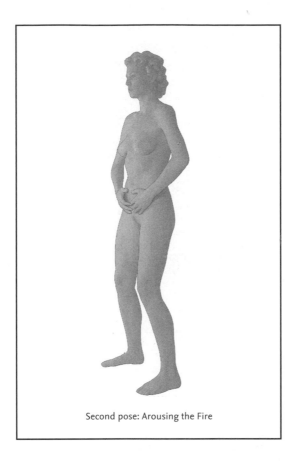

Second pose: Arousing the Fire

Second Pose: Arousing the Fire

In the same standing posture as the first pose, bring your hands to your pelvic area and gently press. At the same time, imagine that the balloon of heat has been pressed into your pelvis. The heat is warming up your pelvis.

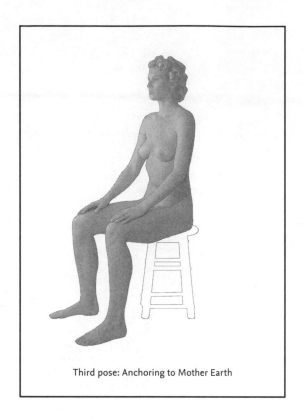

Third pose: Anchoring to Mother Earth

Third Pose: Anchoring to Mother Earth

Sit in a chair with your feet shoulder-width apart. Your feet and legs should be naturally relaxed. With your back upright, gently place your palms on your knees. Tilt your chin downward to allow your eyes to focus on your knees—but keep your eyes closed. Imagine your palms full of warmth, warming your knees as the energy travels downward toward the soles of your feet.

Fourth Pose: Gathering the Energy of Love

On a clean floor or on a moderately firm bed, sit in the lotus position: gently cross—but do not force—your legs. (*Note:* If you find this position uncomfortable, you can continue to sit in a chair as in the third

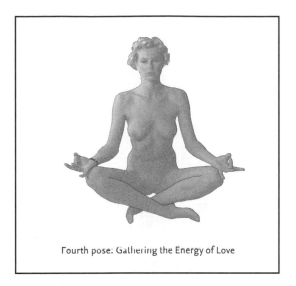

Fourth pose: Gathering the Energy of Love

pose.) The middle finger (the third finger) and your thumbs are touching with the ball of the thumb gently placed over your middle finger nail. Imagine a wave of loving feeling and compassion overflowing in your body.

TIP: Placing the ball of the thumb over the nail of the middle finger is commonly known as the *hand pose of compassion* in meditative practices and Asian religious practices. It induces the integration of our heart and our spirit. This allows the energy of our heart and our spirit to unite and flow freely in a natural expression of our loving and compassionate nature.

Fifth Pose: Tending the Circles of Life

Still sitting in a lotus position with your spine upright as in the fourth pose, bring your palms to your pelvis and gently press them. Breathe slowly without force. Imagine the warmth from your palms radiating into your ovaries. Imagine your ovaries are smiling like the smiling face: ☺

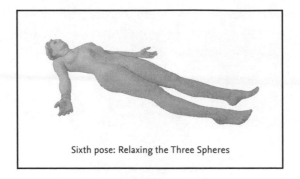

Sixth pose: Relaxing the Three Spheres

Sixth Pose: Relaxing the Three Spheres (Mind/Body/Spirit)

Lie down (on the floor or bed) with both legs straight but separated shoulder-width. Relax both arms at your sides with the palms facing upward. With each breath, especially during exhalation, imagine every single cell and muscle fiber in your body relaxing, from the top of your head to the bottom of your feet. You can begin by focusing on different areas of your head, moving from face, to neck, to shoulder, to chest, to stomach, to pelvis, to lower back, to buttocks, to thighs and upper arms, to legs and lower arms, and downward to your feet and hands.

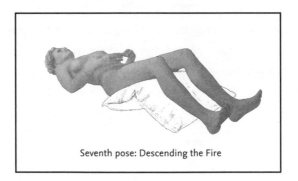

Seventh pose: Descending the Fire

Seventh Pose: Descending the Fire

This is not unlike the second pose, but now you are lying down instead of standing. Lie down with both feet approximately shoulder-width apart and allow your body to be completely relaxed. If it is more comfortable, you may put a soft pillow underneath your knees. Bring your hands to the front of your pelvis. With your elbows on the floor or on the bed, place your palms so that they are facing your pelvis. Again, imagine that there is a small balloon of warm air in this space between your palms and your pelvis. This warm air is penetrating your pelvis.

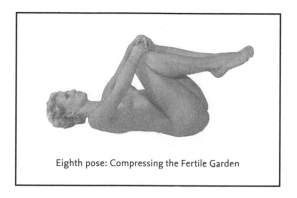

Eighth pose: Compressing the Fertile Garden

Eighth Pose: Compressing the Fertile Garden

Bending your knees, bring them upward toward your pelvis. Grab your left hand with your right hand, creating a lock on your knees and legs. You will feel some pressure in the front of your hip joints and perhaps even on your pelvis. This pressure should be present but not painful. Imagine your abdomen flattening and your hips relaxing more with each exhalation. This should bring your knees slowly and naturally closer to your pelvis. Breathe deeply and slowly. This pose creates pressure in your reproductive system through your pelvis, especially the fallopian tubes and the upper part of your uterus. It increases the stimulation and blood flow into the area.

Ninth Pose: Opening the Gate of Phoenix

Continuing from the eighth pose, bring your arms down to both sides of your body with the palms facing upward. Let your bent knees gently open to either side. The hands assume the hand pose of compassion. Continue to breathe slowly and naturally. Imagine a wave of loving feeling and compassion overflowing in your body. This pose helps to relax your cervix and the lower part of the uterus.

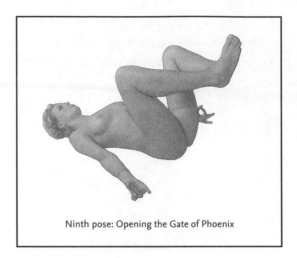

Ninth pose: Opening the Gate of Phoenix

Tenth Pose: Opening the House of Conception

Bring your legs down. Then bend your knees and allow the soles of your feet to face and touch each other. Take care that you allow your knees to fall naturally to either side without force. Assume the hand pose of compassion and place the back of your hands on the inguinal area next to your genitals. As you do this, imagine that the inside of your uterus is like the floor of a tropical rain forest. It is mossy, thick, warm, damp, and rich with nutrients and all the ingredients for life. Any seed that falls onto this floor will germinate. This pose relaxes your entire reproductive system and allows it to open.

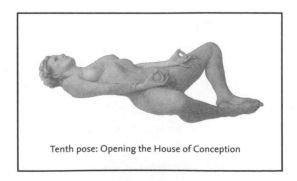

Tenth pose: Opening the House of Conception

Reducing Stress Through Meditation: A How-to Guide

Stress is a funny thing. You feel stressed because you can't get pregnant, yet that same stress decreases your fertility. Research findings prove this to be true. Every day I see women who are exhausted by the pressure of trying to juggle their work and home life while doing whatever it takes to get pregnant. What's the solution? Eliminate stress? Just be happy?

Easier said than done—but not impossible, if you are willing to change your way of thinking. To give you an example from my own life: In college I worked in a supermarket as a grocery bagger. It wasn't exactly a glamorous job, and at five dollars an hour, I certainly wasn't getting rich. But I decided that as long as I was there, I was going to make the work enjoyable for myself. And I did. I overcame the boredom so completely that instead of watching the minutes tick away on the clock, the hours flew. How did I do this? By challenging myself to have fun and laugh at life.

Here's what I did. I first made sure that every single grocery item went into the right place in the bag. I thought about the placement of each item, how to make sure the jam and the butter were in no danger of being smashed together. I thought about how to place the tissues at the top so that they wouldn't be crushed. There's an art to packing groceries, just as there's an art to doing anything in life.

As I got better at placement, I got quicker. When I had learned what I needed to do, I could complete the task in minimal time. That took care of one challenge. Then I needed another to keep my job interesting. So I looked at the checkout aisle next to mine and slowly figured out how to bag for two aisles at once. And that is what I did.

Did anyone tell me to do this? No. Were there a lot of people who thought I was crazy for working so hard? Yes. But I knew I wasn't crazy or even working too hard. I was simply enjoying my work by making it challenging for myself.

The point is that you make your life the way you choose. It's all in the way you look at things. Recently a woman came to my office for treatment. She was having difficulty conceiving and had come to me after

Women's Voices

"It had become very stressful. During the time I was trying to get pregnant, I always ovulated on the weekend. My husband was managing a restaurant, and that was his busiest time. It got to the point where his performance was definitely inhibited by the stress. I'd get angry. I felt I was doing everything I could and I just needed him to be there."

several unsuccessful attempts with IVF. One of the things she mentioned during our conversation was how stressful her work was. I asked her what she did, and she explained her work and all the politics that were involved, including a new boss who wanted all the power. She was thinking about quitting, but she was worried about finding another job. Try as she might, she could not see a way out.

I held up a silver dollar and told her to look at it. What did she see? She might have thought I was crazy, but she dutifully described the building and the icon. Then I flipped it over to reveal the face that was previously hidden. There it was—the lesson. If she only looked at one side, she would never know what was on the other. In her situation, she saw her boss as trying to steal her power. But there was another way of looking at it. From what my patient said, she had responsibility for many employees. What if the boss was trying to share that responsibility rather than steal her power? Was that not a blessing in disguise? Did she ever think that her boss was just trying to do her job? I shared with her an important lesson I've learned through the years: If someone wants to become more proactive, help them. Don't struggle.

The truth is that you can never really control the outcome of anything. Don't jump in and force things. Changing the way you think can change everything—maybe not all at once but a little at a time. Sometimes that is all you need. Be a solution and not a problem.

With all the stresses in life, something has to give. Stress will affect you. You can choose to be happy, enjoy your life, and challenge yourself. When you stop challenging yourself, challenges will soon find you. Wouldn't you rather have the power to choose?

Women struggling with infertility encounter stress that I cannot as a man even begin to imagine. I do know this: Life is precious; every moment is a treasure. At the end of the day, you cannot lose your spirit, your mental perspective. Your soul comes first.

Stress thrives on chaos and uncertainty. That is why it is so important to have a plan when dealing with your fertility issues. You need to understand the whole fertility field so that you can make choices. You must anchor and ground your spirit before you take one more step on the path. You must ensure your intimacy with your partner if you are in a relationship. You must gain perspective and try to put your mind at ease. One of the best ways to do this is through the practice of meditation.

In the broadest sense, meditation is the training of our mind and our spirit. People tend to think that meditation is just sitting still. But it can take many forms, and it can be done for a wide variety of purposes. The Chinese have different techniques for meditating. So do many other cultures. There is standing meditation, where you squat slightly. There is walking meditation. There are meditations practiced in solitude and meditations practiced in groups, with drumming and dancing. The possibilities are endless. But the number one goal of meditation is always the

Women's Voices

"It was horrible. I would run to work, and then make some excuse so I could run to the lab to get my blood tests. I was doing these rounds of IVF, and no one knew. So then I would go back to my work and my life and pretend everything was fine, even though my hormones were so completely out of whack that I had no idea what I was doing. . . . And then I'd find out I wasn't pregnant. Again. And the whole cycle would start all over."

same: learning how to let go of control and any mental distractions and worries you might have.

For some reason, meditation is daunting to a lot of people. So many times I hear: "But I don't have time to learn it," or, "Someday I will devote the time to study meditation." In reality, meditation is simple. Anyone can do it without extensive training. Yes, you can learn it now!

The first thing you need is time. Not a lot—half an hour in the morning and half an hour at night is ideal. If you can't do that much, even five minutes will help. Do it before others wake up or when things quiet down at night. Unplug the phone and then get into a lotus position on the floor. Remember when you were a child and sat on the floor in school with your legs crossed? That's the lotus position. But if that is too complicated for you, just sit on a comfortable chair or couch. Sit straight and relax—but don't lounge. Sit upright and then drop your shoulders. Close your eyes and allow your breathing to be natural, slow, and deep.

It sounds deceptively simple, doesn't it? But when you do this simple process, you are starting to do something wonderful: you are starting to quiet your mind. I can hear you protesting now: "Quiet my mind? How can I do that when all these thoughts keep coming into my head?" Of course those thoughts are there. They will always be there, and when you begin to meditate, you will be hearing them even louder than you do at other times when you are busy with work, home, and family. Is this a contradiction? No. You will hear these thoughts more intensely because you are allowing yourself to hear them. They'll be different thoughts than the ones you think when you are busy. When you are quiet, empty spaces

---

Women's Voices

"Before I went for treatment, I thought traditional Chinese medicine was on the fringes. But it was a whole different experience, not at all the cosmic spiritual stuff I was expecting. It *was* spiritual, but it was also very available. It changed my thinking and my life."

enter between your usual thoughts. When this happens, other thoughts emerge.

The important thing is not to force your thoughts. And don't struggle to vanquish them. Let the thoughts in; let them sit. Just keep relaxing, and be conscious of your breathing. Breathe deeply and slowly. The more you breathe, the more these thoughts will flow. Let them in, welcome them—and then let them go. *Let it be.* That is the very essence of meditation. Let your thoughts do what they want to do.

> *Attain the utmost unoccupiedness.*
> *Maintain the utmost stillness,*
> *And do not interfere with all the things*
> *That rush together in activity and grow luxuriantly.*
> *Then you can see how living things flourish*
> *And renew themselves.*
>
> —FROM *THE COMPLETE WORKS OF LAO TZU,*
> TRANSLATION AND ELUCIDATION BY HUA-CHING NI

What if the thoughts are negative? That's all right, too. We all have bad thoughts, worrisome thoughts—that's part of our everyday stress. While you are meditating, the key is not to dwell on them. It's as if someone is across the street and says hi to you. Maybe you look at him and maybe you acknowledge him with a wave. But you do not cross the street to start a conversation with him. What happens if the person is persistent and crosses the street to tell you a story? Then just listen. Be there, be present—but don't engage in a dialogue. After a while, the person will simply move on. So it is with your thoughts. All you need to do is wave them on as they pass—and keep breathing.

Some people use other ways and techniques to induce a meditative state. These include mentally counting sheep, chanting mantras, reading affirmations, or touching and counting beads. Buddhists traditionally chant while meditating as they count a string of beads, passing it through their fingers. Whatever helps your mind to relax is what you should do. When your mind is calm, your body can follow. Eventually, you will find yourself in a state much like sleep, because your body is not requiring energy to run around and do things. This is what we call being in the

> **TIP:** Eight Treasures is a comprehensive exercise program that is part of the Ni family tradition. The exercises incorporate strength, meditation, stretching, and balancing. They are very helpful in developing better concentration and reducing stress. For more information, you can visit www.taoofwellness.com.

meditation zone. Your energy can now be used to repair and nourish your body.

Think of a dam: When the dam is open, the water is flowing. Close the dam, and the water becomes a trickle. Meditation closes down the energy that flows through your body during the course of your everyday activities and allows your body to replenish it. When you are quiet, several things happen: your heartbeat slows down; your nervous system relaxes; your nerve impulse level decreases. Now your energy can go to places that need maintenance and repair—places like your ovaries so that you can have better egg quality. It's a simple equation: stress reduces fertility; meditation reduces stress; less stress equals better fertility.

I encourage you to take this time for yourself so that you can allow the energy to go back into your body. Replenish yourself. How do you know when you are doing it right? It's not something you can really measure. There's no destination in meditation. Like everything else in life, it's a journey. If you are feeling relaxed and quiet, and paying attention to your breathing—you're on the right road. It does become easier as time goes on. It's like riding a bicycle. After a few times, it will become second nature to you. With continued practice, your body will actually know how to relax more quickly. You will find yourself going to a place where you can't really sense your own body. Then the healing can truly begin.

EXAMINING YOUR
READINESS TO
HAVE A CHILD

If we know the Mother, we may know her offspring.
Know the offspring, yet stay with the Mother.
And the essence of life will never be exhausted,
Even though your body be dissolved.

——FROM *THE COMPLETE WORKS OF LAO TZU*
TRANSLATION AND ELUCIDATION BY HUA-CHING NI

There are many philosophies in the world, each one an attempt to make sense of the life we see around us. I was raised in the Taoist tradition. When people ask what that means, I tell them it's learning to live in harmony with nature. That may sound like a simple idea, but it's not. Why? Nature doesn't want to live harmoniously with us. If you don't believe me, think of the natural disasters we must overcome in this world: hurricanes, typhoons, earthquakes, fires . . . and that's just the start. There are animal attacks, people fighting, and competition for resources. The list goes on and on.

Above all else, there is war. Not just in the sense of people fighting with one another but in nature fighting against itself. You could say that nature is constantly at war and peace, as the tai ji symbol beautifully illustrates. Taoists accept that the world is always living in chaos, searching for balance. That doesn't stop us from trying to find some organization within it.

Take the seasons. I live in Los Angeles now, where people joke that seasons don't exist. But if you carefully observe nature, you will see that there is a certain rhythm to the weather pattern. Within all of these sunny days, there are patterns of change. I see these subtleties as I look around me. Perhaps there's a little more rain, a little less dryness; an earlier fire season, a later summer. To be sure, these are small changes that are not necessarily dramatic unless you are a cyclist or an in-line skater at the beach, where it is easy to feel the wind shifting directions or the light changing color. But there are definitely seasons in Los Angeles. Every day has changes, and every day is a little different from the one that came before it. You just have to look to see it.

Too often we move through life on automatic pilot, unaware of the changes taking place around—let alone within—us. But each day is brand new. And each day, you, too, are new. Your energy is different; your body is different; your attitude and your spirit and all the things that make you who you are are different.

When you are trying to get pregnant, it's important that you recognize these subtle changes. You must learn to read the signs in your body and know what it is trying to tell you. If you are having difficulty achieving your goal of motherhood, you are in essence fighting nature. That's why it's so important to arm yourself with as much knowledge as you can about your current health and your health in the past. Only then can you start to see the patterns in your life. Once you do, you can see more clearly the path you need to take.

Women's Voices

"I approached getting pregnant as if it were a marathon. I wanted all aspects of my life to work together. Nutrition, exercise, the spiritual . . . I think you need to trust your intuition about what your body needs. Dr. Dao's method was harder and took longer. But ultimately, it got me to my goal."

But tai ji (the union of yin and yang) is never simple and never perfect. So the contrary can also be true. There are times when not having a child is truly compassionate and loving. You must look deep within yourself and examine why you want to be a mother. Then ask yourself a few more questions: Will you be able to take care of a child? Do you have the resources, both emotional and financial? This kind of soul searching is especially important if you have never had a child. No one can tell you what to do. You must look hard for the answers within yourself.

I cannot do the soul searching for you. But I do know you cannot just automatically think: I want to get pregnant, no matter how well or ill I feel. In my practice, I have seen too many women who are desperate to have a child simply because they feel they are getting older and their time is running out. But consider this: If you feel old now, how will you feel when that child is ten? If you push yourself too hard to get pregnant, what will that do to your health? Can your constitution handle pregnancy well? Will you recover quickly? Will you be able to breast-feed? And more importantly, is this pregnancy going to injure your health?

You should also take the time to consider what kind of health and genetics you might be passing on to your child. To illustrate my point, a few years back, a woman came to me for treatment. Her genetic profile of her family had many problems: a history of breast cancer on both sides of the family, early death of parents, obesity, alcoholism, depression, heart attacks. . . . This was her legacy. Even so, I was taken aback when she told me outright: "I am not going to have my own genetic baby, because my genes are bad. I do not want my child to suffer the consequences of what I already know." She truly understood what it was to be compassionate and loving. For her, that meant not having her biological child or even pursuing a donor egg alternative or adoption. She decided not to be a mother because she knew with her family history that there was a good chance she wouldn't be around to care for her child. That was an amazing level of self-awareness.

The pull of motherhood is strong. But you must try and break through your little envelope and start seeing things in the broader sense of universal energy. We live a dualistic existence, not unlike stepping into two canoes with one leg in each, trying to sail through life. When the water is smooth, we are fine. When the water gets rough, it threatens to pull us apart.

In today's society, most women work. Many cannot or will not adjust their working lives so that they can put in the time needed to relax, plan, and improve their health before they try to have a child. Some women even approach getting pregnant like an intense work project. This might be good in some cases, but for most this approach is far too stressful. In fact, it can actually decrease your fertility potential. A common scenario in my clinic is seeing a woman who is not physically healthy yet who feels she must get pregnant right away—despite the drawbacks her health might pose for her pregnancy and child. Then there are women who cannot accept that they are aging. They continue to stimulate their ovaries with drugs and engage in IVF procedures until they either get sick or their partner leaves. I understand the longing to have a child. I believe we should have the right to good reproductive health care and support. But being a mother is a gift, not an entitlement or a right. It is a privilege and an honor, and it shouldn't be rushed into blindly.

Maybe you have thought about these things. Maybe you haven't. While you are preparing your body for pregnancy, take a moment to think about the true meaning of love. If you are having problems seeing the light for yourself or making decisions about the steps you will take, you may want to talk to your close friends or seek counseling from mental health professionals. I have worked with many professionals who are excellent at helping people sort things out. They are out there, eager to help you. You are definitely not alone.

Being pregnant and having a child are among the most profound experiences in life. They wake you up in ways that nothing else can. But they also require sacrifice. The truly wise know that you cannot have everything. First, examine your heart. Then, if you seek a child, seek that child with all your heart. And know that if you receive the gift of motherhood, your life will never be the same again.

What Is Your Fertility Potential?
A Questionnaire

As Taoists, we believe that we embody the formal energies of our ancestors. We carry their genetic information, their personalities, and their energetic legacy. We have similar ways of thinking about events in our life. Our environments might be different, but we are all still dealing with basic life issues such as shelter and food, material goods, and comforts. Sometimes it seems like we are repeating life over and over again—what came before is and will always remain a part of us.

This principle takes on particular meaning when you are trying to have a baby. Your health and your lifestyle are certainly key components in determining your fertility potential. But your mother's health, habits, and history, especially when pregnant with you, also play a huge role. The more you know about her, the more you can know yourself. That is why the first part of the questionnaire includes questions about your mother. The remaining questions are about your past and present health history and your lifestyle.

I have designed this questionnaire to give you some relative idea of where you stand with your fertility potential; it is by no means an absolute measure of your fertility. Answer each question to the best of your knowledge and check the box that best applies to you. If you do not know the answer to a question or have never had a specific test or procedure, simply do not answer the question.

Once you have finished, enter the numbers next to the box you have checked in Column A and place their sum in the box marked Total. Then subtract this number from 100. The result is your final score.

Part One: Your Mother's Medical History

questions	answers	column a
1. Did your mother ever take diethylstilbestrol (DES) during her pregnancy with you?	Yes ☐ (2) No ☐	

questions	answers	column a
2. Did your mother ever take any other medications or recreational drugs that are known to cause birth defects during her pregnancy with you?	Yes ☐ (1) No ☐	
3. Did your mother drink alcohol throughout her pregnancy with you?	Yes ☐ (1) No ☐	
4. Would you say your mother's health was good during her pregnancy with you?	Yes ☐ No ☐ (1)	
5. Were you born prematurely; that is, more than a few weeks before your actual due day at forty weeks?	Yes ☐ (2) No ☐	
6. At the time of your birth, were you underweight?	Yes ☐ (1) No ☐	

Part Two: Your Childhood Medical History
(*Note:* The questions in this section refer to the time
before the onset of your first period.)

questions	answers	column a
7. How would you describe the general state of your health throughout your childhood?	Good ☐ Fair ☐ Poor ☐ (1)	
8. Did you ever have diseases or sicknesses during your childhood with high fever that lasted more than five days?	Yes ☐ (1) No ☐	
9. Were you frequently tired during childhood before the onset of your first menstruation?	Yes ☐ (1) No ☐	

Part Three: Your Menstrual History

questions	answers	column a
10. How old were you when you had your first period?	15 or younger ☐ 16 or older ☐ (1)	
11. During your adolescence, would you say your periods tended to be regular; that is, occurring every month?	Yes ☐ No ☐ (1)	

questions	answers	column a
12. Thinking now about the past two years, how many days would you say, on average, your period lasts?	3 or less ☐ (1) 4–6 ☐ 7 or more ☐	
13. Would you say you frequently use pain medication during your period?	Yes ☐ (1) No ☐	
14. Would you say you frequently experience menstrual cramps that last more than two days?	Yes ☐ (1) No ☐	
15. Would you say you frequently experience vaginal bleeding—or "spot-ting"—in between your periods?	Yes ☐ (1) No ☐	
16. Would you say you frequently experience pain during ovulation that requires the use of pain medica-tion?	Yes ☐ (1) No ☐	
17. Would you say you experience night sweats or hot flashes occasionally?	Yes ☐ (5) No ☐	

Part Four: Your Medical History

questions	answers	column a
18. How old are you now?	28 or younger ☐ 29–35 ☐ (5) 35–38 ☐ (10) 39 or older ☒ (20)	
19. Have you ever had any of the following procedures: cervical biopsy, cervical conization, laparoscopy, laparectomy, appendix removal, tubal surgery?	Yes ☐ (2) No ☐	
20. Have you ever been diagnosed with anemia, urinary or bladder infection, vaginal yeast infection, uterine fibroids, polyps, hypothyroidism, rheumatoid arthritis, or osteoarthritis?	Yes ☒ (2) No ☐	
21. Have you ever have been diagnosed with fibromyalgia, Lyme disease, chronic fatigue syndrome, or diabetes?	Yes ☐ (2) No ☒	

questions	answers	column a
22. Have you ever had a blood test on the second or third day of your cycle with FSH levels above 10? (You need not answer if you have never had the test or if you are not sure of the result.)	Yes ☐ (5) No ☐	
23. Do you know if your fallopian tube or tubes are blocked based on the result of a hysterosalpingo-gram? (You need not answer if you have never had the test or if you are not sure of the result.)	Yes ☐ (5) No ☐	
24. Based on a laparoscopy, have you been diagnosed as having endometriosis?	Yes ☐ (3) No ☐	
25. Do you have a history of pelvic inflammatory disease?	Yes ☐ (3) No ☐	
26. How many pregnancy losses have you had (total of all miscarriages and abortions)?	0 ☐ 1 ☒ 2 ☐ (1) 3 or more ☐ (2)	

Part Five: Your Lifestyle

questions	answers	column a
27. Do you have a past history of overconsumption (more than 14 drinks per week) of alcohol that lasted more than six months?	Yes ☐ (1) No ☐	
28. On average, how many alcoholic beverages do you currently consume in one week?	0 ☐ 1–5 ☐ 6 or more ☐ (1)	
29. Within the past two years, have you ever used any recreational drugs such as cocaine, heroin, or other controlled substances?	Yes ☐ (1) No ☐	
30. Have you ever smoked or been consistently exposed to secondhand smoke?	Yes ☐ (1) No ☐	
	Column A Total	

For your Relative Fertility Potential Score, subtract the total in column a from 100. write your answer here:____78____

What Your Results Mean

Your Relative Fertility Potential Score gives us an idea of how your fertility potential might have been compromised. It does not mean that you cannot get pregnant. It is just a means by which to measure the relative difficulty you might encounter.

Good Fertility Potential Score	90–100
Fair Fertility Potential Score	80–89
Moderately Compromised Fertility Potential Score	70–79
Severely Compromised Fertility Potential Score	69 or less

If your score indicates moderately or severely compromised fertility, or if you are thirty-five or older, you should seek the help of a reproductive medicine professional right away. If you are older than thirty and have been trying to conceive for one year unsuccessfully, you should also seek the help of a reproductive medicine professional. If you under thirty and have tried for more than two years without success, you should see a reproductive professional.

Women's Voices

"I was arrogant, but mostly ignorant. I thought, if I am young on the outside, then I must be young on the inside, too. I'm good to go, I kept telling myself. And meanwhile, my ob-gyn was showing me a graph with a steep cliff. And there I was, falling off at thirty-five."

The Myth of Endless Fertility

As you can see from the questionnaire, age is one of the most important determinants in how easily you can expect to get pregnant. As you age, fertility decreases. Your fertility is usually the strongest in your late teens—admittedly, not usually the ideal time for pregnancy. In your twenties, your fertility begins to moderately decrease. By the time you are in your thirties, your fertility enters a new phase. It decreases dramatically after age thirty-five. Adding diseases, illnesses, poor lifestyle choices, stress, and genetics, your fertility erodes even further.

We do not have an eternally high fertility potential. Time chips it away, bit by bit.

Am I saying there is no hope? Life itself is hope. It's like a dream or a wish that comes true. Right now you are wishing you'll get pregnant and have a viable pregnancy with a healthy baby at the end of it all. There's nothing wrong with that wish, because you should always, always have hope. Yes, you might be getting older; you might have health issues. It doesn't mean you give up. Just be sure you balance that wish with reality. It's all right to push hard as long as you know what you are fighting against. The questions you have about your fertility potential have just been answered in a brief way. It is a start. The real stakes are still to come.

But for now, your bags are packed. Hopefully, you're mentally, physically, and emotionally prepared for the road that lies ahead. Before you move forward, let's not forget the most important thing of all: love. After all, love is what is driving your journey. It's love for the child you hope to welcome into your life, love for the ability to become a mother and extend your energy to the next generation. And then there is the love you feel for your husband or your partner or for whomever is sharing this journey with you.

Nurture that love. It will be your ultimate strength.

Before we begin the next part of our journey to fertility, I would like to leave you with something that has been in my family for many, many generations. It's called an affirmation, which is a spiritual tool used to guide you through certain passages of life when you need to affirm your faith and hope. It's like a chant, really, to remind yourself that your body is a little universe ready to release the energy you need to cut through the entanglements that surround you. Calling forth this energy helps you move forward.

"The Golden Light" comes from the *Workbook for Spiritual Development* written by my father, Hua-Ching Ni. I have adapted this affirmation for fertility purposes. As you prepare for your fertility journey, may it bring you peace and light.

"The Golden Light": Dr. Dao's Invocation for Fertility

As the Universe divides, Heaven and Earth are spontaneously manifested.
Clear, light energy becomes the Heavenly Realms.
Dark, heavy energy becomes the Earthly Realms.
In my being, the energy of Heaven and Earth unite.
My being is the temple of the Universe.
I cultivate the way—the way of storing the energies of Heaven and Earth.
My mind is the infinite Heaven.
My mind is peaceful and open, and let all willing beautiful spirits engage me.
My body is the vast Earth.
My body is full of vitality, nurturing and ready for life.
My ovaries are the golden sunrays, which warm up my entire pelvis.
My uterus is a rain forest, where all lives grow and perpetuate.
My uterus is a house; it is comfortable, cozy, relaxed and ready to receive.
My spirit is true.
My wishes are genuine.
May the Universe bring comfort and peace to all lives.
May the Universe select me to carry on the spirits of mankind . . . by conceiving and giving birth to willing spirits . . . to fulfill my destiny as the Universal Mother.

Part Two

ON

THE PATH

If you hope to expand
You should first learn how to contract.
If you hope to become strong
You should first understand weakness in yourself.
If your ambitions are to be exalted
Humiliation should always follow.
If you hold fast to something
It will surely be taken away from you.
This is the operation of the subtle law of the universe.
The law of the universe is subtle,
But it can be known.
The soft and the meek can overcome the hard and the strong.
The true strength of a country or a person is not on the outside.
Just as fish cannot leave the deep
One must never stray from one's true nature . . .

—FROM *THE COMPLETE WORKS OF LAO TZU,*
TRANSLATION AND ELUCIDATION BY HUA-CHING NI

THE TWENTY-EIGHT-DAY
FERTILITY PROGRAM

Harmonious relationship can be illustrated
By the cycle of the seasons
Which produces rain and dew
At exactly the right time.

FROM *THE COMPLETE WORKS OF LAO TZU,*
TRANSLATION AND ELUCIDATION BY HUA-CHING NI

And so the Monkey King took the monk's hand and started on his long jour-
ney to the West to bring the Buddhist scripture back to China. Along the way,
he and the monk were joined by two of the most unlikely traveling companions—
a humanized pig and a priest. They battled their way toward their destination
for fourteen long years.

You are more fortunate than the Monkey King and his companions. All I am asking of you is twenty-eight days to follow a program designed to optimize your fertility potential through a careful selection of foods, exercise, and spiritual reflection. Why twenty-eight days? Twenty-eight days is the length of the ideal menstrual cycle (which also roughly corresponds to the lunar cycle). Regulating your menstruation is the single most important task you face when you are trying to get pregnant.

Your menstrual cycle is composed of many separate yet interconnected processes, all of which must happen in synchrony before you can actually become pregnant. In simplest terms, there are four basic phases: menstrual, follicular, ovulatory, and finally, luteal. In Chinese medicine, we view this cycle as not unlike our four seasons: cleansing, growth, peaking, and withering. Here is how these four phases unfold over the course of one cycle:

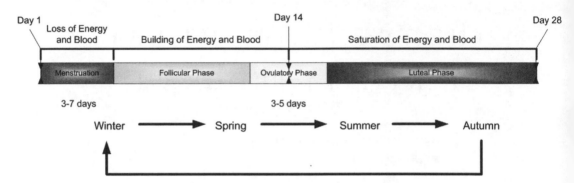

Winter is the season of cleansing, contracting, and ending. It is when the storms arrive. The harshness of winter inhibits the activities of many living things. Plants shed their remaining leaves and branches and stand dormant; animals hibernate or become quiet. The land is frozen. *Menstruation* is very much like the energy of winter. The shedding of the uterine lining, the contracting and cleansing of the uterus, and the quietude of female hormone activity mirror the quietude of winter. Just as there are seeds and organisms under the earth preparing to sprout and thrive once the weather warms, so there are follicles within your ovaries, waiting for the signal to grow.

In spring, plants begin to sprout, adding new leaves and branches. The earth is filled with new life, with hope and beginnings. The *follicular phase* is very much like the energy of spring. It's the time between menstruation and ovulation, the start of a new fertility cycle. The follicles gradually grow, until one follicle stands out—like a bride ready to meet her groom.

Then comes summer, when life is at full bloom, reaching its most abundant level of energy. The *ovulatory phase* is like the summer season. This is the moment when the follicle grows to its maximum size and maturity before releasing its egg. But first, there are last-minute surges and tensions in your body. Luteinizing hormone (LH), which has been synthesized and secreted within your brain by your anterior pituitary gland, must work in concert with other hormones such as follicle-stimulating hormone (FSH). There is also estrogen, which triggers ovulation. This surge of hormones not only signals the ovaries to release the egg but begins the process of nourishing the uterine lining (endometrium) to provide a receptive place for the embryo.

In autumn, the earth continues to be filled with activity. The leaves begin to fall and the temperature drops as the land prepares for winter. The wind is stronger and the air turns dryer. This is the season of harshness. It's a time when the earth readies for the final shedding of leaves and branches. The *luteal phase,* the time between ovulation and menstruation, is much like autumn. It is a time when the uterine lining continues to build up before the final shedding in menstruation.

For simplicity's sake, I have pared these four separate parts down into two. By combining the menstruation and the follicular phases—or, if you will, winter and spring—you arrive at the first phase of the Twenty-Eight-Day Fertility Program. This is the phase before ovulation. It starts on the first day of your period and continues through the fourteenth day.

On the fifteenth day, you will start the second phase of the fertility program. This is the ovulatory or cleansing phase that corresponds to summer and fall. Stay on this part of the program for at least fourteen days, or until your period recommences. I have created sample menus and recipes for your reference. The key is to vary your food choices rather than just stay with what you like. It's a rule worth repeating: more variety means better nutrition for your body.

Fertility Program Food Menu

Phase One: Days 1–14

This first phase is one of germination and nourishment. For the first two weeks, you will need to eat more foods that can strengthen your egg quality as well as your energy—what the Chinese call your *qi.*

To that end, you will be eating a lot of wholesome grains, as well as high-protein foods. These foods include eggs, meat, and beans. It is important that all of these foods be eaten warm. Refrain from eating raw foods—even raw fruits and vegetables—during this time, because raw foods are harder to digest and require more of your body's energy.

During this phase, you should also make time to exercise. However, the kind of exercise you do depends on how you feel during your period. If you have strong menstrual cramps, it is actually healthier to do more strenuous exercise—fast walking rather than slow walking, or perhaps pedaling a stationary bike—during cramping time only. My one caution is to avoid too much jumping or pounding—that is, no running or jumping jacks. You don't want any retrograde menstruation, which occurs when your menstrual flow goes upward through the fallopian tubes and into the pelvic cavity instead of flowing downward through the cervix and out the vagina. This could potentially create inflammatory activity in your body. Some physicians speculate that retrograde menstruation might be a factor in endometriosis.

If you are very weakened by your menstruation and find yourself feeling drawn or looking pale, it is even more important to eat hot and warm foods and "bloody" foods—Beef bone soup, bone marrow soup, beef chili, and hearty stews. Add root vegetables to your diet, too. Beets and turnips are good choices.

Above all, avoid cold foods, and definitely avoid icy ones. No ice cream and no ice in your water.

In essence, your body is undergoing a cleansing process. Think of it as resetting the clock and starting a new cycle of change. You are gaining a new opportunity to conceive again. Your body is starting fresh. If you think about it, it's no different from the Taoist view that death is not an end, and the end is frequently a new beginning.

Breakfast Choices
1 cup of warm oat bran cereal mixed with 1 cup of warm organic un-
    sweetened soy milk topped with a handful of mixed berries and slices
    of half a banana

COOKING WITH CHINESE HERBS AND FOODS

For many centuries, people throughout the world have used spices and herbs in their cooking, not only to enhance the taste of their food but also for medicinal purposes. In the Chinese culture, cooking with herbs such as jujube fruit (da zao), milk-vetch root (huang qi), Chinese angelica root (dang gui), licorice (gan cao), Chinese yam (shan yao), and many others, have provided families—and women in particular—with strong nourishment. The herbs are usually cooked with meats and seafood in a slower cooking process (like a crock pot) to allow the active ingredients found in the herbs to break down.

These herbs, which are sold by the gram, can be found in herb stores in Chinatown, on the Internet, and sometimes in organic or health food stores like Whole Foods and Wild Oats. If you find that the herbs used in the recipes and food plans throughout this book are too difficult to come by, you can substitute more common spices like fennel, cinnamon, and ginger.

1 cup of warm porridge of brown rice topped with pine nuts, walnuts, and cashews; beverage: 1 cup of hot green tea

1 cup of organic oatmeal cooked with organic rice milk or organic almond milk topped with sliced strawberries and a pinch of ground cinnamon; beverage: 1 cup of hot green tea

3 pieces of lightly toasted multigrain bread spread with 2 tablespoons of organic peanut butter and organic fruit preserves; beverage: 1 cup of warm organic unsweetened soy milk.

3 warm organic blueberry waffles lightly drizzled with fresh organic maple syrup; beverage: 1 cup of warm organic unsweetened soy milk

1 cup of organic whole-grain granola cereal mixed with 1 cup of organic low-fat plain soy yogurt; beverage: 1 cup of warm chocolate-flavored organic almond milk

1 large slice of organic whole-grain corn bread, 5–10 pieces of organic pistachios or macadamia nuts; beverage: 1 cup of warm organic unsweetened rice milk

1 bowl of Chinese Rice Porridge (see Appendix: Recipes, page 239); beverage: 1 cup of hot green tea

Lunch/Dinner Choices

1 medium-size chopped sweet potato or yam, and kale sautéed in chicken, vegetable, or beef broth (see Basic Chicken Broth and Basic Beef Broth, Appendix: Recipes, pages 239 and 241) with sesame oil lightly drizzled on top

1 cup of cooked brown rice with ½ cup of cooked black beans and steamed or sautéed squash or zucchini

1 cup of cooked quinoa or millet (or a combination of both) paired with a combination of sautéed tofu, diced tomato, and chopped green onions.

Sauté the tomatoes first with some olive oil until soft, then add in the tofu and 1 teaspoon of low-sodium tamari soy sauce or Bragg Liquid Aminos (an all-purpose seasoning made from vegetable protein found in most health food stores) plus 1 teaspoon of brown rice syrup. Finish by adding the green onions.

1 cup of cooked brown rice with sautéed green beans and 4–5 ounces of steamed, baked, or grilled halibut or sea bass

Barley Chicken Soup (see Appendix: Recipes, page 240) with any steamed squash and shiitake mushrooms

Barley mushroom soup with carrots and onions, 1 cup of cooked brown rice with sautéed broccoli, water chestnuts, and 3 ounces of sliced grilled or sautéed chicken breast (*Note:* The Barley Chicken Soup recipe on page 240 can be adapted by replacing chicken with 4 cups of chopped mushrooms, and chicken broth with 2½ quarts of organic mushroom broth, available in most health food stores.)

Herbal Organic Chicken Soup (see Appendix: Recipes, pages 240, 241)

Salad of lightly steamed broccoli, steamed chopped green beans, cooked kidney beans, corn, and baked or steamed tofu (can also substitute other protein for tofu)

Phase Two: Days 15–28 (or the first day of your period)

After cleansing comes renewal. During the second phase of this program, your uterine lining builds up and starts to secrete mucus to moisten and make itself attractive to the fertilized egg. Like dough to which yeast has been added, the lining starts to rise and create spaces and crevices in which the egg might implant.

During this phase, you need to eat foods that will help improve the lining, the mucus production, and the blood flow. Concentrate on leafy green vegetables like spinach, kale, and chard, as well as berries, which help to keep the blood running smoothly. As before, avoid icy cold foods.

Exercise in moderation. That means no heavy jumping and no running—for that matter, no activity that would direct the blood flow away from the pelvic cavity. This is the time when the seed is trying to implant. Better bets are Pilates, yoga, and meditative exercises like the chi gong program introduced in Chapter 4.

Breakfast Choices
Protein Shake (see Appendix: Recipes, page 241) served with a warm
  croissant
1 large organic poached egg layered with one slice of organic ham,
  served with two toasted slices of whole-grain English muffin; beverage: 1 6-ounce serving of fresh-squeezed orange juice
2-egg omelet made with spinach, mushrooms, and tomatoes; beverage:
  1 6-ounce serving fresh-squeezed orange juice
1 chicken sausage served with 2 slices of tomato and 4 slices of avocado on
  1 slice of whole grain toast with organic non-dairy spread
Egg and turkey breakfast sandwich: 1 organic scrambled egg, 2 slices of
  turkey breast (hormone- and nitrate-free), 1 slice of tomato, and 3
  thinly sliced avocado sections sandwiched in a whole-wheat English
  muffin
4–5 ounces of soft tofu scrambled with zucchini, green onions, and
  mushrooms wrapped in a whole-grain tortilla; beverage: 1 cup of
  organic soy milk

2 large organic scrambled eggs with a small amount of diced green onions and garlic, sandwiched with two slices of lightly toasted multigrain bread drizzled with 1 tablespoon olive oil; beverage: 1 6-ounce
serving of fresh-squeezed orange juice

Lunch/Dinner Choices

4–5 ounces of wild salmon with 1 cup of cooked grains (brown rice,
barley) served with sautéed spinach

3 ounces of sliced of turkey breast with a side of mashed yams, green
beans, or snow peas and carrots; sliced papaya for dessert

Beets, cooked (preferably steamed) and sliced into a salad of mixed
greens, a handful of pine nuts and walnuts, sliced avocado, and crum-
bled soft tofu or shredded chicken; ½ cup of red or white grapes for
dessert

4–5 ounces of grilled lean sirloin steak with sautéed kale; ½ cup serving
of cherries for dessert

1 cup of whole-grain pasta topped with ½ cup organic meat sauce, with
a side of steamed or sautéed winter squash and carrots

Mussels sautéed with shallots, white wine, and chicken broth served over
1 cup of whole-grain pasta or with 1 slice of whole-grain bread

Self-Help Acupressure: A How-to Guide

During this month-long program, you can further help to improve your
fertility by embarking on a series of acupressure treatments that you can
perform on yourself in your own home. Self-applied acupressure utilizes
the same concepts and principles as acupuncture. Its goal is to unblock the
body's energy meridians. The difference is that you use your hands rather
than needles to stimulate specific points on your body. We will be focusing on those that are tied to your reproductive health. What is good for
your fertility is also good for your general health and well-being.

I have selected four points that you or someone else can massage.
Press these points twice a day, in sequence, morning and night. It doesn't
take that long—just about eight minutes a day. You'll be boosting your
fertility even if you can't go to an acupuncturist.

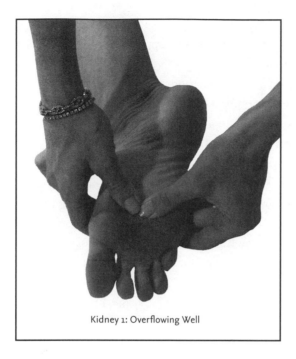

Kidney 1: Overflowing Well

Kidney 1: Overflowing Well

This point is on the sole of your foot. To find it, cup your foot in your hands, with the sole facing you. Now mentally divide your foot into three parts. If your heel is the first part and your toes are the third, the second part is the section that lies right behind the metatarsal joint. It's basically the center of your sole. Place your thumb—the right thumb if you are right-handed, the left if you are left-handed—squarely on this spot. Place your second thumb next to the first and press down hard, wrapping your other fingers around your foot to get some leverage for applying pressure. (Normally, gentle pressure is used in acupressure. However, this one point needs to be pressed harder because the soles of the feet are quite thick and the sensation for this point requires harder pressure.) Press . . . then release. Do this pattern for one minute on each foot.

An even easier way to access this point is to step gently on two small polished round rocks (remember our tribesman friend?). Don't use anything too sharp, because this is a very sensitive point. If you don't have rocks or polished stones, anything oval will do—a small darning egg, a large marble, even a spoon. Stand up and gently apply your weight. Do you feel this point now? In Chinese medicine, we call this the Overflowing Well, because this is where the energy of your body flows to the surface. We consider this a very important point for health and for spiritual meditation. Using acupuncture needles or acupressure techniques on this point can stimulate your entire nervous system and wake up your endocrine system in particular. Anytime you are tired or find that your energy is waning, try this point.

Why is this point so important and helpful to your fertility? Stimulating it helps awaken your body systems and slow down the aging process. It also helps to improve your circulation, particularly blood flow to your pelvic cavity, which in turn can help your egg quality.

Spleen 6: The Gathering of the Yin-Feminine Energy

This powerful point stimulates your female energy and strengthens your reproductive organs. To find it, sit down and cross one leg over the other so that your top leg is at a 90 degree angle. Using your ankle bone as a starting point, lay your four fingers horizontally across your ankle area. Your pinky should be just touching the ankle bone. At the edge of your forefinger, you should feel another bone, located behind your shinbone. Press the tissue

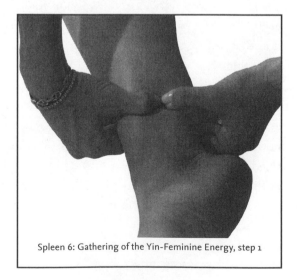

Spleen 6: Gathering of the Yin-Feminine Energy, step 1

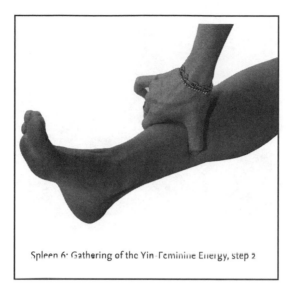

Spleen 6: Gathering of the Yin-Feminine Energy, step 2

area on either side of this bone with your fingers and thumb in the same press-and-release pattern already described. Switch legs and repeat. Or, if you prefer, you can sit in a lotus position and do both ankles at the same time. The sensation should be soothing and extremely calming.

Spleen 10: The Sea of Blood

An easy way to find this point is by sitting on the edge of a chair or couch and placing the palm of your hand on your thigh so that your middle finger is at the edge of your knee. Where your thumb hits on the side of your kneecap is the point you are looking for. Keeping your thumb on this point, straighten your leg and apply pressure using the rest of your hand. Massage one leg, then repeat steps on the other leg.

This point has to do with blood flow. Think of a valve you turn to find the proper water pressure—that's basically what this point is. If your blood flow is too strong, acupressure on this point will reduce it. If your blood flow is deficient, the pressure on the point will release more blood.

When you are young, blood flows richly into your reproductive cavity. Your blood vessels are like newly paved highways. As you age, blood

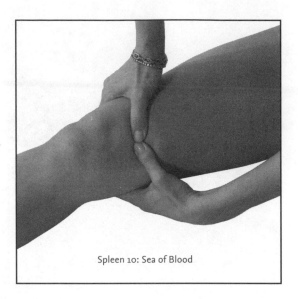

Spleen 10: Sea of Blood

flow lessens. This point improves the microcirculation into your uterus, your fallopian tube area, your cervix, your vagina—all the areas of your reproductive system. When your circulation is better, your health is better—and your fertility is boosted.

Large Intestine 4: Joining Valley

This last point is located between your thumb and your index finger. Open your thumb and index finger wide. Do you see the V? We are looking for the center of that V. As with all other points, press gently. It shouldn't be hard to feel this point. Press for a minute on each side.

This point is good for the immune system and for health in general. In fact, it's one of the strongest and most commonly used points in acupuncture. It's a source of pain relief, including pelvic pain, menstrual cramps, and headache. It's also good for adjusting your nervous system and for bringing circulation throughout your entire body. Unlike the first three acupressure points we discussed, the Joining Valley is not specific to the reproductive system. But with mild massage and stimulation, it can strengthen and revitalize you—and that can only help your fertility.

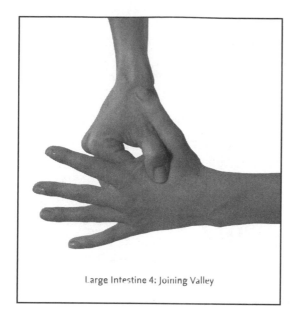

Large Intestine 4: Joining Valley

The Power of Imagery and Affirmation

As part of your fertility program, start imagining. Daydream—come up with a mental picture that conjures up life and growth. Imagine a forest throwing off warmth and moisture. Or imagine a rain forest deep in the tropics. Everything grows there; everything gets fertilized and implanted.

Women's Voices

"I had heard about the mind/body connection, particularly how it relates to fertility. It's about getting centered and peaceful, and letting go of stress. My life is so hectic—I truly believe that's one reason why my egg quality was not as good as it should have been for someone my age. I'm very driven. But understanding how the mind and the body interact has helped me to slow down."

Now imagine that your pelvis or uterus is like the floor of that rain forest. It's warm and spongy, soft and tender. The soil is full of nutrients, so any seed that drops on this floor will germinate and become alive.

The use of imagery to enhance fertility is not new. For centuries in many cultures, imagery methods have been used for having a healthy and strong baby. Today there are integrated mind and body programs that cater to the infertility condition, with imagery designed to help a woman achieve a deeper level of relaxation. More importantly, they help a woman to focus and concentrate on bringing energy and blood circulation to a particular region of her body—for example, the ovaries, the pelvis, or the uterus.

At bedtime or just before you get up in the morning, lie in bed and simply imagine that your body is a receptive, welcoming environment. For ten minutes or so, picture nature springing forth into life. You can also incorporate imagery into the chi gong exercises described in Chapter 4. Try using the pose on page 62 for Opening the House of Conception.

Do's and Don'ts of Fertility

So that's the Twenty-Eight-Day Fertility Plan. But before you continue on your journey, there are a few small reminders. I call them the do's and don'ts of fertility.

Do:

• *Eat green leafy vegetables, fruits, beans, and peas.* These foods all contain large amounts of folate, a nutrient that has been known to help the body make and maintain new cells. Folate helps to prevent anemia, especially around the time of pregnancy and conception. It also helps egg quality, therefore raising your chances of both getting pregnant and staying pregnant.

• *Eat fish and seafood in limited quantity.* As we've seen, eating fish and seafood can be very beneficial. Fish contains omega-3 essential fatty acids, which help reduce heart attack risk, balance triglycerides, and improve blood flow into and around the reproductive system. Be aware, however, of the mercury content in fish, and always follow your local government advisory. If in doubt, take fish oil supplements instead.

• *Eat lean meats and eggs.* Eggs and lean meats contain essential fatty acids and amino acids that are important in reproductive function. They are valuable sources of protein, essential vitamins, and minerals, all of which can make a significant contribution to a healthy reproductive system.

WHAT IS MERCURY AND WHY IS IT SO HARMFUL TO YOUR UNBORN CHILD?

Mercury is a naturally occurring metal that has several forms. It is increasingly found in our food sources and in our environment. Combined with other elements such as chlorine, sulfur, and oxygen, it forms inorganic mercury compounds, or "salts," which are usually white powders or crystals. It also combines with carbon to make organic mercury compounds. The most common one, methylmercury, is produced mainly by microscopic organisms in the water or soil. This methylmercury, which may be formed in water, builds up in the tissues of fish. Larger and older fish tend to have the highest levels of mercury.

When you eat fish or shellfish contaminated with methylmercury, the mercury in your body passes to the fetus and may accumulate there. It can also pass to a nursing infant through breast milk. Mercury's harmful effects that may be passed from the mother to the fetus include brain damage, mental retardation, incoordination, blindness, seizures, and inability to speak. Children poisoned by mercury may develop problems in their nervous and digestive systems, and kidney damage.

Learn about wildlife and fish advisories in your area from your public health or natural resources department. It's a small price to pay for a healthy child.

Consumed in moderation, these foods can help prevent anemia and increase fertility potential.

• *Eat more cooked foods.* Cooking foods can help kill germs and reduce the possibility of catching parasites. By avoiding raw fish like sushi, you can help reduce the risk of sickness as well as improve the absorption rate of your food intake. The end result is better health and increased fertility potential.

• *Eat more warm foods.* Foods warmed to a temperature similar to our body temperature can be much easier to digest, assimilate, and absorb. Thus you utilize more nutrients, which may mean better fertility.

• *Eat dark chocolate.* Eating a small amount of dark chocolate can lift your mood. When your mood is positive, your body functions are more efficient. Happiness and less stress mean better fertility. Stick to chocolate with higher cacao content (50 percent or above).

• *Drink green tea.* Green tea is a powerful antioxidant. It inhibits cancer cell growth and lowers LDL cholesterol (elevated levels of LDL can have an adverse effect on cardiovascular health). Cholesterol is a fat- and hormone-building substance that is naturally produced by our body. But cholesterol levels can also be affected by the foods we eat. There are basically two kinds of cholesterol: the "bad" form known as LDL (low-density lipoprotein) and the "good" form known as HDL (high-density lipoprotein). The latter improves microcirculation in your body. That's important to the development of both your eggs and your uterine lining. (For more information about cholesterol in general, check out the website www.americanheart.org.) Limit yourself to two cups of green tea per day.

Don't:

• *Follow a high-protein diet.* While a high-protein diet can control weight in some instances, it is not healthy, especially when you are trying to have a baby. It puts an unnecessary burden on the liver, pancreas, and kidney systems by forcing them to work hard to digest and break down the extra protein.

• *Follow a high-calorie diet.* Although a popular practice before running a marathon or engaging in strenuous physical activity is to consume large amounts of calories, this raises blood glucose and puts an unnecessary burden on your metabolic system.

• *Follow a high-fat diet.* This fad in weight loss is unhealthy in the long run. Not only does it burden your liver, it also interferes with proper estrogen production in your body, which can negatively influence the proper functioning of the endocrine system and your ability to develop normal, healthy embryos.

• *Eat refined sugar.* A rush of sugar into your bloodstream is the best way to throw off your blood sugar balance. A compromised metabolic system can increase inflammatory activities in your body—in turn, reducing the chance of embryo fertilization and implantation.

• *Eat foods high in sodium.* Excessive salt intake not only raises blood pressure, but it also causes water retention throughout the body. Excessive intracellular fluids can weaken proper functioning of the reproductive system and decrease fertility.

• *Follow a low-fiber diet.* Fiber is an important food source that improves digestion and nutrient absorption. Better absorption of nutrients means better nourishment to your reproductive system. Following a diet low in fiber not only decreases motility in the intestines, but it also reduces the absorption rate of food nutrients.

• *Eat foods just because they look and taste good.* Good taste and appearance don't necessarily mean good health, especially when the foods in question are laden with fats and sugar. Some of these foods also contain additives such as artificial flavors and colors.

• *Favor particular foods.* A wide spectrum of foods is required to provide your body with the nutrients necessary for optimal reproductive function. Don't limit yourself to eating only certain foods.

• *Overdo consumption of convenience foods.* Not all convenience foods are bad. But most of the time, convenience eating means fast foods, which tend to be higher in fats, sugar, and salt, and have reduced nutritional value—not a good idea when you are trying to conceive. Be selective.

• *Overeat.* Most of the patients in our clinic who are overweight undergo a weight-reduction program before embarking on trying to get pregnant. Obesity not only reduces the chance of pregnancy, it can also put the health of mother and baby in danger during pregnancy. Obese patients have higher rates of complications and health problems during pregnancy. If you are overweight, prepare your body before trying to get pregnant.

More Fertility Suggestions

In addition, there are eight areas of your life that you can work on during this fertility program that will enhance the likelihood of conceiving and supporting a healthy pregnancy and baby.

1. Stop Smoking

Smoking is not just terrible for your health, it has strong adverse effects on fertility potential in both men and women. Active and passive smoking increases the time it takes to get pregnant, increases the loss of ovarian follicles, brings on earlier menopause, increases the odds of miscarriages, and increases genetic defects in babies. In men, smoking is associated with decreased sperm count, motility, shape, and function. If you stop smoking, you may improve your natural fertility potential right away.

2. Sleep Well

Consistently getting eight hours of deep, uninterrupted sleep per night is essential to optimal fertility. Good sleep is not beneficial just for the body but also for your hormones and reproductive health. Many women today are not getting the sleep they need. There are many factors that can interfere with our ability to get a good night's sleep. Work- or family-related stress, stimulation before bedtime, ailments such as allergies and pains, noise level in the bedroom, and uncomfortable bedding can all contribute to sleep problems. I always recommend that my patients go to bed no later than 10:00 P.M., with thirty to sixty minutes of relaxation before bedtime. During this presleep time, you should avoid intense discussions, watching television, or engaging in stimulating brain activities. Quiet the house and dim the lights to prepare your body for sleep.

3. Reduce Work and Work-Related Stress

In this competitive capitalistic world, most people have to work long hours under great stress. Your body detects if you are under a lot of work stress and reduces your chances of getting pregnant. It's the body's way of protecting you. Aim for no more than a forty-hour work week with a maximum one-hour commute to minimize stress and maximize your chances of getting pregnant. On the other side of the equation, no work or no social activities can also cause great stress. When there is too much time to obsess about fertility issues, the increased mental stress can further reduce fertility potential.

4. Manage Stress about Getting Pregnant

Infertility is stressful and stress reduces fertility. It is a catch-22 condition. When you become deeply involved in your pursuit of pregnancy, life is no longer as fun or spontaneous. Relationships begin to develop friction. Your social life diminishes. You get depressed. You are unhappy with yourself. This infertility thing becomes all-consuming when it doesn't have to be.

It is not always possible to eradicate all the stress associated with trying to get pregnant, but you can manage it better. The first step is to have a plan, especially when it comes to fertility treatment. A treatment plan should include time for natural conception, time for natural treatment, and time for the number of cycles of IUI (intrauterine insemination) or IVF you will do maximally if you choose to incorporate them.

Develop a support group of close friends or relatives who you can talk to on a regular basis. Join an infertility support group. See a therapist. Your doctors can also help you to devise a plan of action. Aim to have a full, productive life as long as it is not overly taxing physically and mentally. A healthy mix of activities and relaxation helps to anchor your mind and emotions. By reducing your stress, you can increase your natural fertility potential.

5. Foster Good Nutrition and Health

Nutritious eating can increase your fertility potential. The key to good fertility is to consume a balance of carbohydrates, proteins, and fats. Do not skip meals. Chew well, and do not rush through meals. Eat plenty of green vegetables and fruits. Eat an ample amount of foods that contain fiber. Drink plenty of water—up to five 8-ounce glasses a day—and avoid sweets, alcohol, and caffeine.

6. Increase Intimacy

When we are closer with family, friends, or pets, this can increase our sense of well-being and increase fertility potential. Spending more time with friends and with your partner, and socializing without sacrificing your sleep, can bring you closer to your inner self. You will be happier, more content, and more relaxed. This sense of well-being can increase your fertility potential.

7. Embrace Nature

A serene natural environment such as a park, a beach, or the mountains can provide a wonderfully soothing healing power. Taking more time for vacations and relaxation in nature can help you to rejuvenate and refresh your body and soul. This can increase your vitality and enhance your fertility potential.

8. Practice Visualization, Affirmation, and Meditation

Positive thinking brings good energy to your body. A relaxed body will be more fertile than a tense body. Check out the many different books and CDs on meditation techniques and relaxation in your local bookstore. Incorporate the chi gong and meditation exercises in this book into your daily routine of self-care. Be good to yourself and those you love. Believe in the goodness of the universe.

SIGNS IN

CHINESE MEDICINE

Look at it, but you cannot see it.

Because it is formless, you call it invisible.

Listen to it, but you cannot hear it.

Because it is soundless, you call it inaudible.

Grasp it, but it is beyond your reach . . .

But in the mystical moment you see it, hear it and grasp it. . . .

FROM *THE COMPLETE WORKS OF LAO TZU,*
TRANSLATION AND ELUCIDATION BY HUA-CHING NI

The workings of the universe form the basis of Chinese medicine. We observe nature so that we might see how these same processes work inside our body. We can frequently note changes in the inner workings of the body by examining its outer parts. Your body tells a story. If you look carefully enough, it is constantly telling you a story of your state of health. The Chinese believe that any changes in your body will be reflected externally by specific symptoms and signs. By observing changes on your tongue, on your face, or in your pulse, and by analyzing other symptoms you might have, a Chinese medicine professional can develop a good idea of your fertility potential and the nature of your problems. Obviously, not all fertility problems can be diagnosed in this manner. That is why a combination of diagnostic workups using both conventional and Chinese medicine provides a much more comprehen-

> ### Women's Voices
>
> "This system of medicine is centuries old. It makes perfect sense to me. Chinese doctors know more about our bodies than Western doctors do. I have great respect for the method. I believe in the naturalness and longevity of it."

sive view than one method alone. In this chapter, I will introduce you to the world of Chinese medicine diagnosis.

If you came to me with fertility concerns, the first thing I would do is feel your pulse on your left and right arms, look at your face, examine your tongue, and then ask you about symptoms you might have. I would evaluate your history and analyze any conventional workups you might have had. But your tongue, your pulse, and your face would provide me with most of the information I would initially need to know.

The Tongue

Let's start with the tongue. Think of all the things it can do. It is helpful in chewing and swallowing our food. It plays a critical part in helping to form the sounds of our speech. It is the chief organ of taste, and it helps us determine what and (ideally!) how much food to eat. Think of how birds and frogs use their tongues to catch insects and how dogs and cats use their tongues for grooming and to show affection.

To Chinese medicine practitioners, the tongue is a truly remarkable organ, not just because of what it can do but because of what it can show us in terms of a person's general health and well-being. This part of the body is very rich with blood, and the color of the blood shines very close to the surface. In addition to being highly vascular, the tongue is richly supplied by nerve and taste receptors. Salivary glands are standing by just underneath the tongue to moisten it in order to mix with food so that food begins to be broken down before it gets to the stomach. Since saliva contains water, electrolytes, mucus, and enzymes, it can change the appearance of both the tongue and its coating, depending on physiological changes taking place within your body that might change the composition or consistency of the saliva. By observing your tongue, I can see how your whole body is functioning and detect imbalances in different systems of your body.

In Chinese medicine, we divide the tongue diagnosis process into three distinct parts. Each part has a story to tell us. In the first part, which we call the tongue proper, we look at the tongue itself. We analyze the size of the tongue compared to the opening of the mouth and look for any telltale signs of teeth marks, which may indicate edema or swelling in your body. Lacerations or ulcerations of the tongue may indicate that your body is fighting some kind of inflammation. The color of your tongue tells us a lot about the strength of your body, especially regarding blood production, blood flow, and the immune system. A normal tongue is pinkish-red with a certain shine or luster. When the tongue appears pale, it may be a sign of anemia or of a weakened body. When it is red, it may indicate hyperactivity in different systems of the body. When the tongue has a tinge of purple, it might be an indication of pain, congestion, or blockages in the body.

The second aspect of the tongue that we look at is its coating. A normal tongue coating is usually very thin, moist, and clear. A healthy coating means that proper salivary secretions with enzymatic content are taking place in the body. If you have a thick coating, it could mean that there is an imbalance in your digestive system. If your tongue coating is thick with a dirty white color, it usually means your digestive system is suffering from an overgrowth of bacteria in your intestinal flora, mostly candida.

Candida is a fungus that belongs to the yeast family. It grows in our mucous membranes—mostly in the mouth, esophagus, stomach, intestines, and vaginal areas—along with many other microorganisms that help us break down foods, toxins, and bacteria. But when candida is out of control, it can cause different kinds of fungal infections, especially in patients whose immune systems are compromised. One of the most common yeast infections is *Candida albicans,* but there are many others. If this is a chronic situation, it means that you are either overeating or that the body is not able to assimilate the food you are putting into your body and your body has become inflamed, causing dysfunction in the intestines.

If the tongue coating is thick and yellow, this might mean that some form of inflammatory or infectious activity has been going on in your lower urinary tract or reproductive system. At the opposite extreme, if the coating is stripped so that the tongue is mirror-smooth or is dry or peeled, this indicates dehydration of your system, in which case essential fluids need to be replenished. A peeling coat or a cracked tongue indicates depletion of essential fluids or malnutrition.

The third aspect of examining the tongue is by regional analysis. Different areas of the tongue represent the functioning of different regions of the body. The tongue is divided into four regions: front, middle, back, and sides. The front part of the tongue reflects the organs and systems of the upper part of the body, mainly the respiratory and nervous systems. Any changes in this area might point to the common cold, flu, upper respiratory infections, sleep disorders, or even changes in mental state. The middle part of the tongue reflects the organs in the center of the abdomen, mainly our digestive system. Changes in this region of the tongue can be an indication of trouble in the digestive and absorption functions of the body. The sides of the tongue represent the flank or side areas of the body, mainly the liver and spleen. These organs have to do with the detoxification and circulation functions of our body. Changes in this region can indicate fluctuating toxicity levels in the body. A darkening of this region can also mean poor or changed circulatory function, which can be reflected by symptoms of pain or other discomfort in the body. The back region of the tongue represents the lower portions of our body relating to the bladder, reproductive system, and large intestines. A peeling coating in this particular region can mean endocrine weakness or chronic lower back pain. A thickening or a yellow coating in this region of the tongue can mean constipation, a urinary tract infection, or a vaginal infection.

All this information, just from asking you to stick out your tongue!

The Pulse

The pulse is an extremely useful indicator of the state of your health. Your pulse is basically the palpable sign of the flow of blood and other fluids through an artery. When you are sick, the rhythm and quality of your pulse can change in subtle ways. By differentiating these subtle details, a skilled doctor of Chinese medicine can detect changes inside your body, especially relating to how a disease is progressing and how your body is fighting disease. Understanding such changes becomes useful in determining the best course of intervention or support for your body, and it is particularly important when dealing with infertility issues.

There are a few places where a pulse can be taken. The most common one, preferred by the majority of doctors of Chinese medicine, is your radial pulse located right under your thumb near your wrist on both arms. By placing three fingers across the radial artery and by palpating three distinct depths of the pulse, I can sense imbalances in different organ systems in your body—imbalances that can help me determine what fertility challenge you might be facing.

There are at least twenty-seven major types of pulses. The pulses are classified depending on a combination of characteristics: velocity, width, length, depth, regularity, location, strength, and reaction to pressure. Like the tongue, the pulse under three fingers is further divided into three depths for a total of nine distinct regions on each arm. These regions reflect different parts of the body. Changes in any of these regions can indicate changes in different areas of the body. This is how a Chinese medicine professional detects imbalances in your body through pulse diagnosis.

Reading your pulse for the first time during your menstrual cycle gives me a baseline against which I can measure changes in your subsequent cycles. This helps me to not only determine the course of your treatment, but it also lets me know the kinds of fertility challenges you may be facing as well as the progress of your treatment. For example, a thready pulse, where the width of the pulse is very narrow, like a thin thread, suggests a weakened endocrine state or a lack of blood, a lack of circulation, or a decreased hemoglobin level. A wiry pulse, where the tension of the pulse is tight, might indicate ovulation difficulties or even endometriosis. In this case, pushing down where the flow of the pulse hits my finger feels similar to pressing down on taut tennis racket strings. If you have strong hormones, you might exhibit a slippery pulse, where the pulsating through my three fingers feels like ball bearings slipping through my fingers effortlessly. A certain jumpiness in a slippery pulse may denote a positive pregnancy outcome; this feels not unlike dry beans dancing on a hot pan. By comparing pulses in different stages of a patient's menstrual cycle, I can usually perceive changes and differences that will enable me to adjust my treatments and maximize treatment results.

Pulse reading is also an important tool during assisted reproductive technology (ART), especially when gonadotropins (hormones that stimulate follicle growth in the ovaries) are used to recruit multiple follicles during a cycle of IVF. I can usually recognize whether a patient is doing well with the stimulation long before a hormone test or an ultrasound has been rendered. This is mostly due to the effects of extra estrogen or gonadotropins on the arterial wall. This extra tension of the arterial wall can be detected in a pulse-reading session. Using this information, I am able to work closely with my patient's reproductive endocrinologist to modify the stimulation protocol if necessary to maximize results.

The Face

Your face gives us different clues to your health condition. Take color, for example. If you are pale, it shows anemia or that you are having issues with blood flow somewhere in your body. If your face is red or flushed, it indicates that there is an increased blood flow. We call this "fire rising." In a fertility issue, we see this as a sign that a woman might be going through some perimenopausal symptoms—not an ideal situation if you are trying to get pregnant. If your facial color has a blue-green hue, this might indicate that there are certain areas of your body that have congestion blockages. It also suggests the possibility of pain. A sallow, yellow color is associated with malnutrition, which is more commonly seen in underdeveloped countries.

A swollen face can mean an array of problems. Puffy eyes or cheeks could indicate problems with water retention, and more importantly, problems with your urinary system. Swelling, tightness, and tenderness near your jawline could mean you are clenching your jaw at night while you sleep. Tense sleep is not good sleep. And good sleep is what you need to maintain good hormone secretions to ensure the quality of your uterine lining and your eggs. As we have already seen, a high level of stress is not conducive to good fertility. If your face is emaciated, that tells me your body is in a weakened state. Further tests might be needed to rule out certain conditions like lupus or diabetes. Also, a deviation of the face and eyes—a crooked, asymmetrical mouth or one side of the face dropping down—could be a symptom of a stroke or Bell's palsy.

Even your facial expression reveals volumes about your physical, mental, and emotional health. Are you happy? Sad? Frightened? As you now know, your emotional state can have a great effect on your fertility.

DIAGNOSIS IN WESTERN MEDICINE

Being prepared for hardship
One will not be overcome by it.

FROM *THE COMPLETE WORKS OF LAO TZU,*
TRANSLATION AND ELUCIDATION BY HUA-CHING NI

The Conventional Fertility Workup

When a woman has infertility issues, she usually consults with her gynecologist. The gynecologist then typically recommends and performs a battery of tests and procedures to assess her fertility. These tests should be familiar to most women, whether they are trying to get pregnant or not. They include a pap smear, a pelvic exam, and perhaps a vaginal culture. The gynecologist might also do a few simple blood tests to measure hormone levels. He or she might want to do a pelvic ultrasound to help visualize the

---

Women's Voices

"You can do all the tests in the world, but you can't do anything unless you accurately describe how you feel to someone who is willing to listen."

ovaries and uterus, to see if there are any general abnormalities or cystic structures that might interfere with the implantation of a fertilized egg—for example, ovarian masses, polyps, or cysts.

None of these tests is particularly invasive. In fact, if you were to by-pass your gynecologist and come to me first, I would take the same approach—at least initially. I would ask you to get some blood tests. If you didn't have a gynecologist, I would refer you to a lab. These tests are all part of a preliminary workup. This basic fertility workup is essential to evaluate the whole reproductive system.

If you are a healthy woman in a heterosexual relationship having regular unprotected intercourse, you usually have an 85 percent chance of getting pregnant within a year. If you've been having unprotected sex for more than twelve months without conception; or you are thirty-five years of age or older; or you have irregular menstrual cycles; or you have known diseases that would create difficulties with conception such as tubal diseases, endometriosis, or uterine fibroids, it would be advisable for you and your partner to immediately undergo an initial fertility workup with a health care professional specializing in reproductive medicine. I cannot stress enough the importance of evaluating both partners

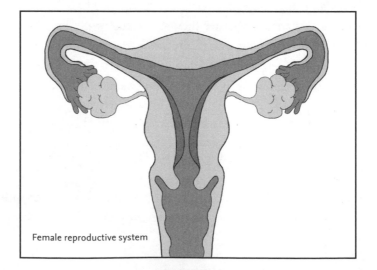

Female reproductive system

simultaneously, since the male partner can account for the problem 50 percent of the time.

For a man, a standard comprehensive semen analysis is usually performed as the first step. For the most part, it involves masturbation and a cup. A fertility laboratory technician will use a computer to scan and visually evaluate the semen specimen.

Not so with a woman. A workup is much more involved because a woman's reproductive system is quite complicated. Usually most of this workup is done by a gynecologist who generally starts by asking about your medical, gynecological, and menstrual history. This is usually followed by a gynecological exam or perhaps a more complete physical to assess your reproductive and physical health. Many women express trepidation about going through all those tests. To put your mind at ease, I'll walk you through them so that you have some idea of what to expect.

Most doctors will ask you to complete a form detailing your medical history. I have one that I use at my clinic (which I have included for your reference at the end of this book). The form may vary from doctor to doctor, but the basic questions are the same. The point is to gather information about any previous illnesses, genetic issues, and current conditions, and to obtain an overview of your menstrual history. You can also expect questions about your current lifestyle, including the use of alcohol, tobacco, or other drugs, and other factors that might affect your fertility.

From there, the doctor will proceed with a physical and gynecological examination. He or she will most likely check your thyroid gland for any enlargement, tenderness, or nodules. A thyroid abnormality could have a strong effect on your fertility potential. Next, the doctor might check your breasts for discharge or secretions, which could be evidence of disease. He will palpate the lower abdomen to check for organ enlargement or masses. The doctor will also examine the uterus to check its size, position, and mobility. This is usually a manual exam. However, he might also order a vaginal or pelvic ultrasound to further evaluate your uterus.

These tests provide a starting place for the doctor to decide whether more tests are needed to identify the cause of infertility. In Western medicine, these diagnostic tests focus on different gynecological anatomic regions. The main areas include the endocrine system, the ovaries, the cervix, the uterus, the fallopian tubes, and any pathology of the peritoneal or pelvic cavity.

Endocrine System

When hormones work together like instruments in a symphony orchestra, they make music. When they do not work together, they make noise and create chaos. The first step in evaluating whether there is an imbalance in your hormone system requires a few simple blood tests. These can include, but are not limited to, thyroid-stimulating hormone (TSH), prolactin (PRL), and follicle-stimulating hormone (FSH), along with your estrogen levels. Blood for these tests is usually drawn on the second or third day of your cycle.

Ovaries

It is often difficult to ascertain the exact cause of ovarian dysfunction, even though it accounts for up to 40 percent of infertility cases in women. That is why so many tests are often required. These tests include the following:

Menstrual History

This history is a chronological description of your menstrual cycles starting from your first period. It covers the time between periods, the length of a typical period, as well as other issues like flow and premenstrual symptoms.

Basal Body Temperature Chart

The hormones in our body can cause changes in our body temperature. By taking your basal body temperature (BBT) every day and charting it, seeing the rise and fall through a menstrual cycle, we can determine the overall functioning of your reproductive hormones. BBT needs to be taken first thing in the morning, before you get out of bed.

Most physicians do not rely on the BBT chart anymore, since it cannot predict the exact time of ovulation. They rely more on the urine LH

BASAL BODY TEMPERATURE CHART

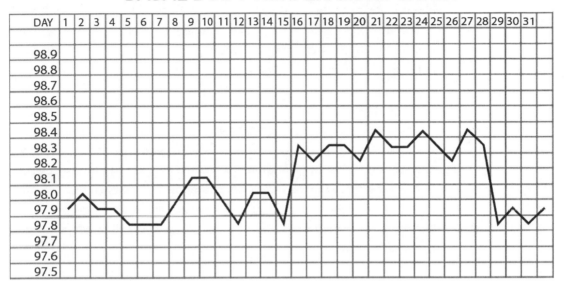

test, progesterone test, and, in some cases, ultrasound. I would argue that the BBT chart does have value in that it tracks the ebbs and flows of the hormones through the entire menstrual cycle. Measuring the basal body temperature during one complete menstrual cycle provides information on the function of the ovary, its follicular development, and the proper secretion of progesterone.

The other advantage of the BBT method is its affordability. All you really need is a chart and a basal thermometer (available in any pharmacy) to track your temperature. When you have a normal ovulation cycle, your BBT appears biphasic—that is, there is a distinct rise and fall of temperature before and after ovulation. When there is no ovulation, there is no appearance of progesterone, which means no rise in your temperature, because rising temperature is directly related to the secretion of progesterone. When we do not detect this rise and fall and the temperature stays the same or just oscillates up and down without an obvious pattern, we call this monophasic.

By assessing your BBT charts for a few cycles, we can begin to see a trend in your overall hormonal and ovulatory cycling. With this information, we can detect subtle problems that can be treated effectively before they become bigger problems. You can make copies of the sample blank BBT chart on page 250 for your own use. In my experience, however, some women find this self-charting stressful. If you find you are one of them, stop doing it. There are plenty of other ways to evaluate your ovulation.

Blood Tests for Progesterone Levels

Progesterone is an essential hormone that is produced after the release of the ovum (unfertilized egg). It causes the lining of the uterus to thicken in readiness for the implantation of a fertilized ovum. By measuring progesterone levels, a physician can determine the adequacy of this hormone in the blood. To make sure you are ovulating, your doctor might order a blood progesterone test. This is usually performed a few days after your anticipated ovulation day.

Tests for Luteinizing Hormone Levels

Luteinizing hormone (LH) levels are a reliable indicator of ovulation. LH significantly increases in concentration in the blood just prior to ovulation. By testing urine for luteinizing hormone levels, it is possible to determine the time of ovulation. Test kits are available for over-the-counter purchase in most pharmacies.

Samples of the Cells of the Uterine Lining (Endometrium)

A healthy and sufficiently thick inner lining of the uterus is essential for a pregnancy to occur. Examining a sample of this lining at a particular time in the menstrual cycle through a hysteroscopic procedure provides valuable information on the development of this tissue in response to hormones released to stimulate its growth and proliferation. It can indicate defects in the different phases of the cycle both before and after ovulation.

Ultrasound of the Ovaries

A physician can use ultrasound to inspect the number of developing follicles (maturing eggs in the ovaries). It may provide evidence that ovulation is taking place or that it's not, depending on the development of the follicle. For example, it may be able to identify a problem with the development of a follicle that would prevent normal ovulation.

There are two common types of ultrasound used in women's health care: abdominal and vaginal. Ultrasound imaging (or sonography) involves exposing part of the body to high-frequency sound waves to produce pictures of the inside of the body. Unlike X-rays, it does not use ionizing radiation. It is used to show structure, movement of internal organs, and blood flow.

Cervical Examination

The cervix is usually checked during a pelvic examination. Your doctor will inspect the cervix for any scarring or inflammation and to assess the sufficiency of cervical mucus secretion. In the past, the cervical mucus was examined, sampled, and tested for possible incompatibility with sperm from a woman's partner via a postcoital test. This involved collecting cervical fluid shortly before ovulation and within hours of intercourse. The sample was then examined for the presence of motile (moving) sperm. The postcoital test is being gradually phased out due to lack of validity.

Uterus

Hysterosalpingography

In hysterosalpingography (HSG), an X-ray is taken of the uterus and fallopian tubes. To assist in the image creation, it is necessary to inject a dye into the cervix so that it fills the uterus and fallopian tubes. This test gives some insight as to the size and shape of the uterine cavity. It also offers information on abnormalities such as fibroids or uterine polyps that may be present, which would affect reproductive success.

Ultrasound

Much like the ultrasound used to examine the ovaries, this test examines soft tissue for abnormalities. It's most often used for the diagnosis of uterine pathologies such as fibroids (myomas and adenomyosis), which may influence fertility. Ultrasound is frequently performed at the beginning of your menstrual cycle to determine available follicles, especially before a drug-stimulation cycle. It is also used during your mid-cycle to help detect and confirm ovulation.

Hysteroscopy

If your doctor cannot be completely certain of what she sees during an ultrasound of the uterus, a hysteroscopy might be ordered. This test involves inserting a camera into the vagina and uterus, where it is used to inspect the uterine cavity. Sometimes water is introduced into the uterus, distending it to enable a better look at the contours of the uterus. This procedure can also be used to view and remove a polyp in the uterus, since polyps can sometimes interfere with implantation of the embryo. A polyp is an overgrowth of tissue in the lining of the uterus. It is like a skin tag or a layer of extra skin. Even though most polyps are small and do not compromise reproductive capabilities, the majority of doctors prefer to remove them so as to rule out any possible interference.

Fallopian Tubes

These tubes collect the ovum (unfertilized egg) after the ovary releases it. The tubes then guide the ovum down to the uterus. The tubes are very important, because they provide the most likely location for the sperm to penetrate and fertilize the ovum. The tubes then provide the fertilized egg with a smooth passage to the uterus to be implanted in the uterine lining (endometrium), where it develops into a fetus. The tubes can often be scarred, obstructing the important connection between the ovaries and the uterus. Scarring, while not the only tubal problem, is the final product of infections and inflammations and a major cause of infertility. Thus it is important to ascertain tubal health in evaluating fertility.

As a Chinese medical doctor, I have great respect for these diagnostic tests. But I would be remiss if I didn't add an observation based on more than twenty years of treating patients. If you've been given information about your infertility that doesn't feel quite right or is confusing, or even makes no sense at all to you, you are not alone. In Western society, we are taught to believe that the doctor is always right. It's hard to speak up when you have questions or concerns. But that's exactly what you must do. If you have a feeling about what's happening or not happening in your body, it's imperative to ask for the care you want. Don't get swept up in fear and anxiety over your diagnosis and allow yourself to make a hasty or pressured decision about your care and about your future. The doctors are here to serve you, but you need to be proactive about your case.

There are a variety of fertility issues that affect women all over the world. Some you're born with; others can develop during the course of your life. The key is to understand what you're dealing with. Some fertility challenges are minor, and if diagnosed correctly, they can be treated very simply. Others are much more serious and require surgery. Realize that no matter what the diagnosis is, you have options.

YOUR FERTILITY MAP

Many words lead one nowhere.
Many pursuits in different directions
Bring only exhaustion.
Rather, embrace the subtle essence within.

FROM *THE COMPLETE WORKS OF LAO TZU,*
TRANSLATION AND ELUCIDATION BY HUA-CHING NI

When the Monkey King set off on his journey, he knew where he was going and what he had to do. How he was going to get there was an entirely different issue.

When you're taking a journey, it's always a good idea to know where you are going. And if you've made it this far, you obviously do: you are heading in the direction of motherhood. That is why you have prepared your mind, your body, and your spirit. But how far are you willing to go to reach your goal? If motherhood is your ultimate goal, would you be willing to contemplate a donor egg or surrogacy if necessary? Are you willing to use assisted reproductive technology (ART) or are you adamant about pursuing a completely natural and drug-free pregnancy? And just how long are you willing to travel? All of these questions must be considered before you can determine the best route for *you* to take.

In order to figure that out, you first have to face your strengths and weaknesses. Up to this point, we have talked about the importance of starting your journey from a place of optimal health and balance. Perhaps you have already started incorporating changes into your daily life to boost your fertility potential. Maybe you've followed the Twenty-Eight-Day Fertility Program and started thinking about your life in a different way. Perhaps you even feel you are in the best health possible. But in Chinese medicine, health is always relative. This is especially true when it comes to fertility health.

No two travelers are exactly alike. One might carry more baggage, one might be older and slower, and one might be more athletic, more energetic, more hopeful. . . . Do you see what I am saying to you? What's more, there are many paths to the same destination. The more you know about your strengths, weaknesses, and tendencies, the better you can choose which path to take.

In order to understand how Chinese medicine works, it helps to know the Western medical approach to diagnosing infertility. In the previous chapter, we discussed the kinds of tests that are used to identify potential problems in women trying to have a baby. Western medicine traditionally focuses on specific factors or challenges. These "challenges" usually fall into specific categories, among them endocrine, ovulatory, tubal, cervical, pelvic, and uterine. Emphasis is placed on finding dysfunctions in specific parts of the body. This diagnostic method is quite effective at discerning the disease-causing mechanism. But by focusing mostly on parts of the body, this reductive method does not concern itself with the patient's ability to fight a disease or overcome a challenge. It also doesn't take into consideration the patient's constitution. This perspective provides only a partial view of the disease process and loses the big-picture perspective that considers a patient's constitution.

Traditional Chinese medicine, in contrast, approaches diseases using a method called *patterns* or *syndromes*. The patterns approach to diagnosis is based on a holistic view that includes both the disease mechanism and the patient's reaction to the disease. We start by taking note of a patient's signs and symptoms. These symptoms are usually placed into contrasting categories: Is the body deficient (reacting weakly to the disease) or in a state of excess (reacting strongly)? Is the condition one of heat (with the body showing symptoms like sweating, fever, or flushing) or of cold (cold hands, cold feet, chills)?

The next step is to determine which organ systems are reacting to the disease. In Chinese medicine, syndromes are named after the organ function system rather than the organ itself. For example, the kidney organ function system dominates the functions of a person's inherited constitution, their reproduction, and their excretion of fluid. Therefore the kidney organ function system can include genetic coding such as DNA; the endocrine system such as the hypothalamus, pituitary gland, thyroid gland, and adrenal gland; the reproductive organs such as the ovaries, testes, fallopian tubes, uterus, and lower reproductive tract; and the fluid excretion system such as the kidneys, bladder, and lymphatic system.

Once symptoms are noted, we seek to find a pattern. For example, *kidney yin deficiency* means that the kidney organ function system is affected, with mostly heat symptoms showing that the body is not putting up a strong fight against the disease. *Kidney yang deficiency* means that the kidney organ system is affected, with mostly cold symptoms that show the body's endocrine function is in a decline.

The liver organ function system tells a different story. This system includes the functions of detoxification, ensuring that all systems of our body are working smoothly. This organ function system can therefore include such organs as the liver, gallbladder, kidneys, spleen, and even the nervous system. *Liver qi stasis* means the body's systems (qi) are not functioning smoothly and the body is strongly fighting the disease (stasis is an excess condition).

Blood stagnation indicates that the blood circulation is not smooth; there is an interrupted flow. The actual flow of the blood may be stagnant or the blood may be too thick.

Phlegm-damp congestion indicates that the body's waste products have caused some obstruction. This waste could be the result of either normal physiological functioning or of infections and inflammations. In infertility, this pattern is frequently seen in tubal obstructions, where fluid or scarring is left from a prior inflammation. It can also be seen in obese patients, where the extra fats in the body are considered a burden and drag the body down, much as waste products do.

These are the five main patterns in infertility conditions in both men and women. The table opposite lists patterns and their symptoms. You will see that some symptoms overlap in the different patterns. Patterns are a relative assessment and are not meant to be an absolute diagnosis. A person can have a mixture or combination of these patterns because the body frequently reacts to a disease condition in many different ways. I have also listed commonly seen clinical conditions in the third column

PATTERNS	SYMPTOMS	COMMONLY SEEN WESTERN MEDICAL CONDITIONS
1. Kidney Yin Deficiency	Early menstruation, scanty menstrual flow, vertigo, tinnitus, lower back pain, blurry vision, frequent visual fatigue, insomnia, many dreams, restless sleep, hot flashes, night sweats, facial flushing, anxiety, dry skin, vaginal dryness, poor lubrication during sex, prone to constipation	Luteal phase defect, elevated FSH, thinning of uterine lining, age-related infertility, perimenopause, poor response to IVF, recurrent miscarriages
2. Kidney Yang Deficiency	Delayed or skipped periods, light, watery, or dark brown menstrual flow, lower back pain, pale face, low or decreased libido, cold hands, cold feet, aversion to cold	Hypothyroid, decreased estrogen levels, poor ovulation, luteal phase defect, poor circulation to the uterus, age-related infertility, poor response to IVF, elevated FSH, recurrent miscarriages, thin uterine lining
3. Liver Qi Stasis	Premenstrual breast tenderness, pelvic or body bloating, easily angered, painful menstruation, prone to constipation, prone to indigestion with distension and gas, insomnia	Fibroids or polyps
4. Blood Stagnation	Clotty menstrual flow, menstruation with pain in the pelvic region, lower back, or legs	Endometriosis, fibroids or polyps, various forms of pelvic inflammations
5. Phlegm-Damp Congestion	Delayed menstruation, overweight, frequent vaginal discharges at times thick and sticky, vertigo, heart palpitations, nausea, abdominal distension, cough, asthma, postnasal drip, nasal congestion, morning sneezing, water retention	Obesity, hydrosalpinx or blocked fallopian tubes, fibroids or polyps, polycystic ovarian syndrome (PCOS)

for your reference. Again, this does not mean a definitive situation but rather a relative likelihood.

Now that you know more about the pattern method of Chinese medical diagnosis, you can start to assess yourself. In the following questionnaire, you will see the five patterns listed across the top. On the left side are questions asking you to identify different symptoms you might have. Each question includes a number(s) in parentheses to indicate which column should be checked. For example, the first question reads: "Are you frequently fearful and scared?" If the answer is yes, you would place a checkmark in columns 1 and 2 (indicated by the numerals 1, 2) under the question. If you don't know the answer to a question, skip it. Continue answering and checking the boxes until you reach the end of the questions.

Once you have finished the questionnaire, add up all the check-marks in the columns. You should start to see a pattern. See which column you checked the most, and whether your total number of answers meet the criteria for that pattern (meaning you have at least 50% of the symptoms). Remember, it's entirely possible that you could have more than one pattern.

What Are Your Patterns?
A Questionnaire

	1	2	3	4	5
	Kidney Yin Deficiency	Kidney Yang Deficiency	Liver Qi Stasis	Blood Stagnation	Phlegm-Damp Congestion
Mind: The state of your mind can influence your fertility. By assessing your current state of mind and emotion, we can better understand which patterns you fit into.					
Are you frequently fearful and scared? (1, 2)					
Are you frequently irritable? (3)					
Are you frequently anxious and overly worried? (5)					

	1	2	3	4	5
	Kidney Yin Deficiency	*Kidney Yang Deficiency*	*Liver Qi Stasis*	*Blood Stagnation*	*Phlegm-Damp Congestion*
Are you frequently in physical pain? (4)					
Body: The state of your body is most important in determining which patterns you fit into. There are many questions in this category.					
Do you frequently have menstrual cycles shorter than 26 days? (1)					
Do you frequently have menstrual cycles longer than 30 days? (2, 5)					
Do you frequently have fluctuating menstruations that can be more than 30 days apart? (3)					
Do you skip periods at least twice a year? (2, 5)					
Do you have light menstrual flow? (1, 2)					
Do you have a large amount of clots during menstruation? (4)					
Do you have menstrual cramps severe enough to require medications? (4)					
Do you have mostly brown menstrual flow? (2)					

	1	2	3	4	5
	Kidney Yin Deficiency	*Kidney Yang Deficiency*	*Liver Qi Stasis*	*Blood Stagnation*	*Phlegm-Damp Congestion*
Do you get chronic lower back pain? (1, 2, 4)					
Do you get vertigo intermittently? (1, 5)					
Do you get ear ringing intermittently? (1)					
Do you get blurry vision intermittently? (1)					
Do you have difficulty falling asleep more than 30 percent of the time? (1, 3)					
Do you wake up frequently at night? (1, 3)					
Do you have many dreams? (1, 3)					
Do you have hot flashes? (1)					
Do you have night sweats? (1)					
Do you have dry skin? (1)					
Has your vagina lubrication decreased? (1, 2)					
Do you have decreased libido? (2)					
Are you prone to constipation? (1, 3)					

	1	2	3	4	5
	Kidney Yin Deficiency	*Kidney Yang Deficiency*	*Liver Qi Stasis*	*Blood Stagnation*	*Phlegm-Damp Congestion*
Are you prone to loose stools? (2, 5)					
Does your face appear pale? (2)					
Are your hands and feet frequently cold? (2)					
Do you frequently have to dress more heavily than others? (2)					
Do you get chilled easily? (2)					
Do you get premenstrual breast pain? (3)					
Do you get strong abdominal bloating premenstrually? (3)					
Are you prone to indigestion with lots of gas? (3, 5)					
Are you overweight? (5)					
Are you underweight? (1)					
Do you have frequent creamy, sticky vaginal discharges? (5)					
Do you get feel nausea intermittently? (5)					

	1 Kidney Yin Deficiency	2 Kidney Yang Deficiency	3 Liver Qi Stasis	4 Blood Stagnation	5 Phlegm-Damp Congestion
Do you get palpitations intermittently? (5)					
Do you have a hard time losing weight? (5)					
Do you cough intermittently? (5)					
Do you have asthma? (5)					
Do you have nasal congestion? (5)					
Do you sneeze in the mornings? (5)					
Do you feel that you are retaining fluid frequently? (5)					
Disease Orientation: Sometimes certain disorders can fit into one or more patterns.					
Do you have uterine polyps? (3, 4, 5)					
Do you have fibroids? (3, 4, 5)					
Do you have endometriosis? (4)					
Do you have blocked fallopian tubes? (5)					
Do you have polycystic ovarian syndrome? (1, 2, 5)					
Do you have luteal phase defect? (1, 2)					

	1	2	3	4	5
	Kidney Yin Deficiency	Kidney Yang Deficiency	Liver Qi Stasis	Blood Stagnation	Phlegm-Damp Congestion
Do you have elevated FSH? (1, 2)					
Do you have a thin uterine lining? (1, 2)					
Are you over the age of thirty-five? (1, 2)					
Are you a poor responder to IVF? (1, 2)					
Do you have hypo thyroidism? (2)					
Have you had miscarriages? (1, 2)					
Total Checked per Column					
	Yes, if greater than 11 checked	Yes, if greater than 10 checked	Yes, if greater than 5 checked	Yes, if greater than 3 checked	Yes, if greater than 10 checked

What Do Your Results Mean?

If you don't have enough checked answers to meet the criteria for any one pattern, it could mean your fertility potential is higher than you might think. That would be the good-news scenario.

Or perhaps you show a clear-cut pattern of responses, indicating that you fit one or more of the patterns. In that case, here are some practical suggestions to help you.

Kidney Yin Deficiency

Kidney yin deficiency in women is indicative of a deficient state of ovarian hormones, namely estrogen and progesterone. Many symptoms such as night sweats, hot flashes, insomnia, restless sleep, dry skin, early menstruation, and decreased menstrual flow can be attributed to this pattern.

Sometimes the answers are simple. By reducing your stress level and bringing more joy and relaxation into your life, you can improve your ovarian hormone function. You can do this by participating in a moderate exercise regimen, taking a class on meditation, and finding time for quiet contemplation and relaxation. By eating more nutritiously, you can also nourish your hormone levels. An adequate consumption of dark green leafy vegetables such as kale, Swiss chard, spinach, bok choy, cabbage, seaweed, broccoli, arugula, collard greens, dandelion greens, mustard greens, and chicory are helpful in strengthening your kidney yin. These dark green leafy vegetables contain good sources of folate, fiber, many vitamins, and minerals that are important in the synthesis of hormones. As a general rule of thumb, the darker the vegetable, the more nutrients it usually has. Eating more astringent types of fruits like berries would be helpful as well. These fruits include raspberries, blueberries, blackberries, gooseberries, boysenberries, and cranberries. Berries are naturally low in calories and filled with vitamin C and flavonoids, which help the body to become healthier and more sensitive to hormone production.

Kidney Yang Deficiency

Kidney yang deficiency suggests broader endocrine deficiencies that go beyond simple ovarian weakness and insufficient production of hormones by the thyroid, adrenal, and pituitary glands. This overall weakness affects how the body functions in the areas of metabolism, cardiovascular circulation, and finally, reproductive function. An aversion to cold and difficulties in ovulation are some of the signs in this pattern.

If you fall into this pattern, you might already be finding yourself craving more warm and cooked foods. Eating a diet that is moderately higher in the animal protein categories can be helpful in stimulating endocrine functions. This can include fish, beef, lamb, turkey, and chicken. Certain spices can also be helpful; try adding garlic, onion, ginger, cinnamon, fennel, black pepper, cayenne red pepper, turmeric, cardamom, chives, cloves, cumin, and paprika to your everyday diet. Engaging in regular moderate exercise activities such as walking, short jogs, stretching, yoga, tai chi chuan, swimming, and using exercise machines can all be helpful in stimulating your blood flow and improving your overall endocrine function. One more tip for frequent travelers: reducing time zone changes can help stabilize your endocrine function.

Liver Qi Stasis

This pattern indicates you might be experiencing a more abrupt cycling of your hormones. This could be due to a temporary spike in your hormone levels or to a greater hormonal sensitivity. For example, some women experience more severe premenstrual symptoms than other women, including moodiness, breast enlargement and tenderness, constipation, food cravings, and insomnia. In most normal situations, the symptoms are mild and manageable, and they do not affect a woman's daily activities. But when this pattern is severe, it is more than discomforting—it might also be an indication of abnormal ovarian functioning such as the presence of ovarian cysts, which put out more estrogen than the body actually needs. This extra estrogen secretion, occurring over a long period of time, can increase the odds of getting uterine and breast fibroids, which in turn can affect fertility potential.

Cooling foods are the best bet for you. You need to eat a lot of vegetables, making sure there is plenty of fiber intake. Drinking more water can also help to balance this abrupt cycling. Including such spices as cilantro, bay leaves, anise, basil, coriander, and mint in your diet can help regulate hormone secretions. Engaging in exercises geared toward focus such as yoga, tai chi chuan, walking, fencing, and dancing can help keep your emotions grounded.

Blood Stagnation

This pattern is used to describe painful conditions. If you have painful menstruation, ovulation, or intercourse, you might have some degree of this pattern. Pains are frequently caused by inflammation, infection, tumors, or elevated secretion of hormones such as prostaglandins that cause unnecessary stronger uterine contractions. If your pain is severe or if you need over-the-counter pain medications, you should consult with your health care professional. But there are other things you can do to help to reduce these pains, especially if you know the pattern the pain typically follows. For example, if you experience severe menstrual cramps each month, I suggest you engage in more strenuous physical activity just before the onset of your period. This has helped many of my patients to manage and decrease the severity of pain. Other effective treatments are acupuncture and herbs. Eating cooked (not raw) foods and decreasing caffeine, sweets, and alcohol intake can all be helpful.

Phlegm-Damp Congestion

This pattern indicates symptoms of excessive mucus production such as sputum, phlegm, vaginal secretion, and mucus in the bowel movement. Mucus is frequently composed of glycoproteins, immunoglobulins, lipids, and waste products. Glycoproteins are blended molecules of sugar and protein. These sugar proteins serve important functions—not just lubricating mucous membranes but also acting as hormone or immune protectors to help fight off diseases. Immunoglobulins are a type of glycoprotein that form the fundamental network for our immune system. Along with lipids, these components protect our mucous membranes, which expose and exchange nutrients with the outside environment. Mucous membranes line the entire digestive tract, the respiratory tract (beginning with the nose), and the vaginal and urinary tracts.

An excessive, sudden, and acute production of mucus suggests infection and inflammation in the body. Chronic and ongoing excessive mucus secretion can mean chronic infections and inflammations, as well as allergies, excess weight, or other metabolic or immune disorders. If you have symptoms of excessive mucus production such as chronic nasal drainage, throat congestion, coughing, asthma, indigestion, gas, bloating, constipation, diarrhea, weight gain, frequent urinary bladder infections, profuse vaginal secretions, or vaginal odor, you have some degree of this pattern.

There are practical steps you can take to help decrease symptoms. First and foremost, address your dietary habits. Avoiding alcohol, sweets, and greasy foods and reducing dairy product intake would be a good way to start decreasing mucus production. Finding out which if any foods are causing allergic reactions in your body can also be helpful. A nutritionist can usually help you figure this out by suggesting an elimination diet plan. An overall reduction of food intake for those who tend to overeat can be helpful. Engage in good hygiene and be sure to make moderate exercise a part of your daily life.

10

DETOURS AND

OBSTACLES

The ancient ones who knew how to live with the subtle
*   essence of the universe were gentle and flexible,*
*   profound and indistinguishable. . . .*
They did not rush into anything, as if fording an icy
*   stream in winter*
They adapted themselves to a circumstance
*   like melting ice.*

—FROM *THE COMPLETE WORKS OF LAO TZU,*
TRANSLATION AND ELUCIDATION BY HUA-CHING NI

Detours do not always occur because there are obstacles on the path. And obstacles do not always cause detours. When you find yourself at a fork in the road and are uncertain which direction to take, you must stop and listen to your inner voice.

There is a guiding voice in each of us that helps us go down the right path. That voice has nothing to do with intelligence or intellect; it has everything to do with your spirit and who you are. Often, your inner voice might contradict what your rational self is telling you. The Monkey King had a solution to such dilemmas: he would pick at his ear, cross his legs, and simply go to sleep.

As it turns out, the Monkey King had it right in some ways. There's no way you can make big decisions about something as close to the heart as fertility without starting from a place of calmness. You are struggling with your fertility now, and you need to clear your mind before you take the next step.

When I have difficulties and the answers don't come to me easily, I take a long hike in the hills of Topanga Canyon, high above the Pacific Ocean. I walk for hours, covering so many miles that my body almost becomes numb. Only then can my mind find solace and inner peace. Hiking in the mountains, feeling one with the earth, I am rejuvenated. My mind becomes clear to the point where I am in touch with who I am and what my purpose is. That is when I realize there is not a lot that is important except for my health, my family, and intimacy with my partner.

Sometimes it is important to take a break from trying to get pregnant. It doesn't have to be long—just long enough to get in touch with yourself. When you hit a snag in your dream of having a baby, don't panic, and don't rush ahead rashly. Above all, know your options. Find a professional guide who has a great knowledge of both natural and conventional medicine. If that's not possible, make sure you have all your bases covered. A reproductive endocrinologist, for example, focuses much of the time on IVF procedures. Such professionals are not a good resource for making an overarching plan with you. That's why you should also include someone either in a mental health profession who specializes in infertility or someone who practices natural medicine with a tremendous amount of experience and expertise in dealing with infertility. That person could be a naturopath, a homeopath, or an acupuncturist with knowledge of reproductive medicine. If you don't happen to know where or even how to find an expert in these fields, there are excellent resources available. (A list is

---

Women's Voices

"It's very intimidating when you're having trouble getting pregnant. You feel vulnerable. In the medical profession, doctors who specialize in fertility tend to make it feel very factory-like or technical. There's not a lot of warmth. It was hard to control things sometimes."

available at the back of this book.) You could visit the Tao of Wellness website (www.taoofwellness.com) for more information.

In the next chapters, you will read the stories of women who faced many obstacles and challenges on their road to fertility. As soon as one challenge was addressed, another seemed to pop up in its place. What all the women have in common is great strength and determination. They were not afraid to keep their minds flexible and their hearts open to whatever life threw at them. This is necessary because getting pregnant is a very intricate process involving many different components and physiological functions of the body.

For starters, it requires a viable amount of good-quality sperm, which must be deposited into the cervix area. It also requires a good quantity of healthy cervical mucus to protect the sperm and assist it on its journey as it swims upward from the cervix, into the uterus, continuing onward into the fallopian tubes. If all goes well, that's where the sperm will meet with a mature egg that has been released from the ovary.

But it's not enough that the egg meets with the sperm. The uterus must have a lining thick and dense enough to be receptive to that fertilized egg so that it can implant itself and begin life. And the uterus itself must be capable of sustaining that growth and the development of the embryo. And so it continues with multitudes of conditions that must be met.

Talk about a complex journey! Even the Monkey King would be daunted. No wonder so many different things can and do go wrong. In fact, when we look at reasons why people have difficulty getting pregnant, we usually see a combination of factors, although there is usually one dominant factor. But as we shall see in the actual case studies in subsequent chapters, what may at first appear to be one fertility challenge often turns out to be another.

In Vitro Fertilization

At least 50 percent of my patients over the age of thirty-five ultimately use some form of assisted reproductive technology that can include IUI (intrauterine insemination) and IVF (in vitro fertilization). Increasing numbers of patients are using TCM & IVF concurrently; others seek my help before attempting these technological processes.

If you know that IVF is going to be part of your fertility journey, I would still advise you to take the time to prepare your body using acupuncture and herbal treatments. It's a good way to maximize your chances of success.

Have you ever gone to Las Vegas and gambled at a slot machine? Even if you haven't, I am sure you are familiar with the way it works. Picture yourself in front of a big quarter machine. The machine allows you to play anywhere from one to five lines at once—your choice. One quarter will give you one line; five will give you all five, or the maximum. When you play only one quarter, you are lowering your chances of a payout, since you only get one line of possibility. If you put in the maximum number of coins, you get in return the maximum odds.

It's the same with IVF. You are gambling, hoping to get a payout—in this case, a viable pregnancy. Now, if you came to me before attempting IVF, I would assess your health status and your readiness to go forward with the procedure. To continue the gambling analogy: Are you going in with one line or with five lines? If I see that you are playing one line— meaning that your health and your lifestyle are not what they could be—I will advise you to save your money. Twelve to fifteen thousand dollars for one IVF procedure is a lot of quarters! But if you are willing to give Chinese medicine even two months to help your body heal and prepare, it can usually bring you closer to five lines. I can't promise a jackpot, but I can certainly increase your chances of winning one.

It seems like such a simple concept. And yet I see women unwilling to invest the time in preparing their body. They feel the need to go ahead right away and have the procedure. The women over forty who come to our clinic feel a particular urgency. To them, two months of preparation seems like an eternity. I understand their anxiety and their feeling that there is too little time to get pregnant as it is. Perhaps that is how you are feeling right now. But I would argue that you cannot afford *not* to take the time to heal your body and become stronger before attempting to conceive by technological methods. You will potentially damage yourself if you push your body beyond what it can do. You must be fully aware of the limitations of your body and any preexisting conditions.

Say, for example, you have a small uterine fibroid. If you start drug stimulation, it's very possible that your fibroid will start to grow and create issues for the very fertility you are seeking to enhance. You may even have to resort to surgery to remove the fibroid, causing more delays in your fertility treatment. Or perhaps you have a history of fibroid cystic breasts. Drug stimulation can increase the density of your breasts, creating the need for repeated mammograms.

There are questions about the drugs used in ART. Recently there was a question about clomiphene citrate (Clomid) and its potential link to cancer. Even though scientists found that infertility patients have a higher risk of cancer, they don't know if it is from the drug or from the condition of being infertile. There was also a research study done in Australia in 1999 that suggested an increase in cancer risk for women with unexplained infertility who use fertility drugs. But subsequent studies have yet to prove an absolute, definitive association between fertility drugs and cancer.

When your body and your health are not strong before you embark on any stimulated cycles with gonadotropins, several things can happen. First, your body may not respond to the stimulation, yielding poor results. Second, your endocrine system becomes even more tired, meaning you run the risk of creating perimenopausal symptoms. We have already mentioned the danger of aggravating existing medical conditions. But for every time you do a round of IVF without success, your chances of conceiving in subsequent cycles decrease.

Suppose you are one of the lucky ones who manages to get pregnant and deliver a healthy baby at a later stage of life using modern technology. There's still the simple element of exhaustion to contend with. IVF and motherhood can take a lot out of you. Your energy goes down along with your endurance. The quality of life is difficult at times. And yet there is no real way to track the effects of delayed motherhood, mainly because the women who manage to have children at an older age are reluctant to complain, having attained their dream of having a child.

These are all things you must think about before entering the world of ART. Pregnancy is only a process, much like IVF. You might get pregnant using IVF, but that doesn't ensure a healthy pregnancy. It certainly doesn't ensure a baby—ask any woman who has gotten pregnant by IVF only to see the pregnancy slip away in the first critical weeks.

You must be prepared before having IVF. But most IVF doctors do not have the opportunity or time to teach you how to do this. Their primary goal is to carry out the procedure with minimal complications, and for the most part, they do that very well. As a practitioner of natural medicine, I do not perform IVF, even though I work every day with IVF patients and their doctors. I know my limitations. I can't stimulate the development of multiple follicles; I cannot implant embryos. Chinese medicine is not an interventional medicine. It is a rejuvenating and re-plenishing medicine. As a Chinese medical doctor, I cannot separate re-productive health from a woman's overall health. It's a message that bears repeating: better health means better fertility.

I personally believe that IVF is incredible technology. It's a wonderful tool that has helped many women to achieve their goal of having a baby—and certainly, there are many situations in which ART is neces-sary. But I also think we need to use it judiciously and wisely. I see too many women who have attempted this highly invasive procedure over and over again. Some have done IVF five, even six or more times, each time flooding their bodies with the powerful drugs and hormones that are necessary parts of the process. It's very intense and demanding on your body and health, to say the least. You really need to evaluate your body and be in good health for IVF. And yet women don't usually do this. The

Women's Voices

"Sometimes I wonder if we've become this kind of society where there's a cure for everything. I don't think most people realize it. I re-member my dad saying, 'If it's money or something, I would be more than happy to pay for the IVF treatment.' I appreciated it but told him to forget the money. IVF isn't just like going in and having a shot, no matter what people may think."

irony is that many jump too quickly into the world of IVF, often skipping a simple first step like insemination that would be much less invasive for their body, not to mention considerably less expensive. IVF should be for the woman who has exhausted other less invasive procedures and who truly needs it.

It all comes back to the importance of having a plan. If you skip steps and don't take your time, you will have pain in your life—with or without a baby. Be strong, be determined, but above all, be wise.

Part Three

INFERTILITY
CHALLENGES

If you hope to expand
You should first contract
If you hope to become strong
You should first weaken yourself.
The law of the universe is subtle,
But it can be known.
The soft and the meek can overcome the hard and
    the strong.

—FROM *THE COMPLETE WORKS OF LAO TZU,*
TRANSLATION AND ELUCIDATION BY HUA-CHING NI

11

OVULATION

By the time I was twelve, I was diagnosed with dermoid cysts on both ovaries. My left ovary was removed; fortunately, they were able to save my right one. Several years later, I started having severe stomach pains. They found more cysts. This time, they couldn't salvage much. Only the tail end of my remaining ovary was left, and all signs were that it was nonfunctional. Within days, I started having hot flashes and other symptoms. According to my doctor and the blood tests, I was already in perimenopause. Right away, I was started on progesterone and estrogen. The doctors said I would never have children. I was all of twenty-one. . . .

Dr. Dao told me from the start that there was about a 0.5 percent chance of getting pregnant. And that was enough for me. That 0.5 to me was my egg. I knew there was something left. The hard part had always been trying to find someone with the wherewithal to get it.—Rita

Ovulation is probably one of the most important aspects of fertility. Women who have difficulties with ovulation account for up to 15 percent of all infertility cases (factoring in the male partner). Frequently, I come across women who do not ovulate consistently on time. Sometimes this translates into irregular menstrual cycles; sometimes, however, the menstrual cycle can be perfectly consistent. For this reason, it is important to pinpoint the exact time when you are ovulating.

A useful tool is a test called LH surge, an over-the-counter urine test (more commonly known as an over-the counter ovulation kit) that helps predict the timing of your ovulation by measuring the presence of luteinizing hormone (LH), which is secreted by the pituitary gland located beneath your brain. This hormone plays a critical role in triggering ovulation.

Another tool is the basal temperature chart (see page 250). Although not a good predictor of ovulation, it does offer a retrospective look at how hormones are secreted throughout your menstrual cycle. In addition, pelvic ultrasound can be used as a way to confirm ovulation.

Many women have only a vague idea of when they actually ovulate. They know that ovulation usually occurs around the thirteenth to the fifteenth day of a normal menstrual cycle, but they are less certain of the signs that often accompany it. Some of these signs or symptoms may include increased vaginal mucus and discharge, lower abdominal twinges, increased libido, and nipple and breast sensitivity. It is important to know both when you are ovulating and how you feel during that time. Fluctuations in timing and symptoms could be the first sign of decreasing fertility.

Even if you ovulate like clockwork every fourteen days, you might still be facing an ovarian challenge. The reason has to do with your luteal phase, the time between ovulation and the beginning of your period. Ideally, this phase is fourteen days. But for some women, the luteal phase is much shorter. This is not a good sign. For one thing, this shortened luteal phase suggests a potential problem associated with the production of progesterone, the hormone that keeps the uterine lining strong and receptive. A shortened luteal phase means that the progesterone levels declined prematurely, resulting in earlier menstruation. Since progesterone is largely secreted by the corpus luteum, the part of the ovum that is left behind in the ovary after ovulation, this can also indicate a problem with the quality of the egg. Poor egg quality can mean problems with the uterine lining, resulting in less overall receptivity to the fertilized egg and a lessened chance of getting pregnant.

Moreover, if your progesterone level starts to drop and you start having a ten-day luteal phase instead of one that lasts fourteen days, your uterine lining sheds prematurely, leaving your fertilized egg an insufficient amount of time to get to your uterus and make a home there. This seems to be a common issue in older women who we see in our practice.

Conventional medicine addresses this issue by prescribing progesterone supplementation. But merely putting women on progesterone supplements in these situations does not necessarily improve the chances of pregnancy. In fact, if you look at this problem from the bottom up, you will realize that the issue is the egg quality, because sufficient progesterone should be secreted by the corpus luteum. If there is a deficiency of progesterone secretion, chances are the egg quality is also weak.

How do we assess whether you have an ovarian challenge? After confirming whether you are ovulating or not, the next test is to assess your relative ovarian reserve. Blood tests for FSH and estrogen levels on the second and third days of your menstrual cycle are frequently used to give us an overall idea of your ovarian reserve. Another way is to stimulate your ovaries and endocrine system with medications to see if your ovaries get "tired" under duress (we measure this by testing FSH levels before and after stimulation).

For example, in the clomiphene citrate challenge test (CCCT), a drug called clomiphene citrate is used to stimulate your ovaries. A reading of your FSH level is taken before and after stimulation. If that number rises after stimulation, your ovaries are probably not very strong, or they have a relatively weak ovarian reserve. There are other challenge tests as well, using different ovulatory agents but measuring similar outcomes. These ovarian reserve challenge tests give us relative—but not absolute—results that provide some idea of whether your ovaries are functioning normally.

Ovulatory challenges or dysfunction may be severe enough to actually prevent pregnancy. Or they might simply be one of many factors or challenges a woman faces in her journey toward fertility. In the case of at least one woman I treated, the outcome was nothing short of miraculous.

Rita's Story

I first met Rita in February 1999. She was thirty years old and had a sad history of many different health problems. But her biggest problem concerned her ovaries.

At twenty-eight, I married my boyfriend. I knew what the doctors had said— that I would never have children. But now I was starting to see everyone having a family and building their lives. Naturally, I got very depressed until I finally decided to do something about it. I did a lot of research and started asking my doctors a lot of questions. For so long I had been told I was perimenopausal. But what exactly did that mean? And why were they treating me as if I were already in menopause? The doctors told me that I wasn't functioning normally for my age. According to them, I was well on my way to menopause.

I wasn't swallowing it. I wanted a family. They shut me off. So I started looking for an open door.

Rita had very little ovarian tissue left. When I saw her, she had been having extremely irregular periods for several years. She'd also been on hormone replacement therapy (HRT) because of her severe menopausal symptoms. She had experienced weight gain, severe mood swings, hot flashes, and other symptoms that bothered her a lot. But she was determined to get pregnant and had already sought treatment at a fertility clinic.

I went to a big fertility expert who took me off the drugs I had been taking and put me on an estrogen patch. The idea was to try me on shots of Pergonal, an ovarian-stimulating hormone. I think now they were just trying to pacify me. They knew it wasn't going to work—that's why they didn't come at me full force with medications and procedures. And sure enough, it wasn't long before they suggested a donor egg. The shots hadn't worked and neither did the patch. So I found a donor. I was happy with that because I finally believed that my getting pregnant wasn't going to happen any other way.

Aside from her ovarian issues, Rita was slightly overweight, and she had asthma and difficulty breathing. There was a family history of diabetes. Rita was also highly allergic to many kinds of substances.

And then the donor backed out. That was very depressing, to say the least. I started hoping again that there might be some other way for me to get pregnant without a donor egg, but the doctors were very clear: it wasn't going to happen. When I still didn't accept it, they thought I was in serious denial and gave me the name of a therapist. I saw her for one full year. And all that time I was still convinced I would get pregnant.

I went to see another doctor. I liked her from the start. The first thing she said was: "If you are still trying to get pregnant, why are you on all this estrogen?" I was grateful that someone at least acknowledged that I hadn't given up hope. She told me there were healthier ways to ensure that I was getting enough estrogen. She also said there was an acupuncturist who could work with me to get me healthier. And if he could help to get me pregnant . . . well, that would be great, too. Unlikely, but great.

You would have thought I'd have jumped on it. Here I was spending thousands of dollars on patches and shots, so why was I suddenly so reluctant to try something else? I thought this was just another kind of medicine that didn't work. My husband was the one who convinced me. He figured I'd tried everything else. Why not try this one last thing?

I went to see Dr. Dao. I was used to being put on a table and told by doctors there was nothing they could do for me. But Dao pulled at my wrist and looked at my tongue. I was taken aback, sitting in his huge office, on this Chinese barrel-like seat, completely surrounded by books. This was a serious place. And this was a serious man, warm but very real. I could tell he felt bad about what I had gone through and that he wanted to help me.

On that first day I saw a woman who was very sensitive and highly emotional. Her FSH level had been fluctuating greatly, with numbers usually associated with women in the perimenopausal stage. Because of her unique situation, I decided that our main focus would be to see if we could reduce her hot-flash symptoms and maybe even reverse her ovarian aging. As we talked more about her history, I began to see that her sensitivity might work for her. You might call it the silver lining in the cloud. I felt she might respond very strongly to acupuncture treatment. If that were the case, we might even be able to get her to ovulate. Obviously, I told her there were no guarantees. The plan was to work on her treatment for about three months to see how she'd react and respond.

Despite being a complete needle phobic, I agreed to try the acupuncture twice a week. But I didn't want to take any herbs. With all my allergies, I didn't want to put anything foreign into my body.

The first treatment went extremely well. In fact, Rita's period started three days afterward, which was not as surprising as it seems. Because of the hormones she had been taking, she had been experiencing anovulatory cycles—bleeding even though she was not ovulating at all.

But by the next few visits, Rita had developed headaches and nervous tension after her acupuncture treatments. Interestingly, to her, the head-aches seemed like a positive sign. She told me that in the past, when she was younger and menstruating regularly, she would have headaches once a month around the time of her period. To her, these postacupuncture headaches felt just like her hormone headaches. She also felt tired after the treatments, which was to be expected, given her extreme sensitivity.

At that point, I advised her to get strict about her diet. I told her to avoid refined sugar and to increase her protein intake. I also told her to exercise every day. Soon her headaches began to decrease. What's more, she started to feel twinges in the ovary area after the acupuncture treat-ments. But these positive signs were tempered by new information: Rita had considerable bone loss, much greater than other women her age. Such loss in a young woman, if not caused by medication, is usually associated with low estrogen levels. In Rita's case, the cause was not clear. Her over-all health and her endocrine system were not in the greatest shape.

But by the fifteenth day of her cycle, Rita told me she'd been feeling really good after her acupuncture treatments. She felt comfortable and relaxed; and what's more, she described feeling actual twinges in her uterus and in her ovary and pelvis.

I decided that I would buy ovulation kits—lots of them. One day, I came in to see Dr. Dao and told him the stick was blue—I was ovulating! I had only been seeing him for a month.

This was something of an amazing change, because Rita hadn't been ovulating at all during all of the hormone replacement therapies she'd had. But she was sure she was ovulating now, because she had a very strong pelvic ache after her treatment. In fact, after her treatment she went to buy another ovulation test. The test confirmed ovulation. What's more, her hot flashes were down to zero.

So with the blessing of her doctor, Rita went off all of the hormones she had been taking. Other than feeling a little tired at night, her energy was good—a vast improvement over what it had been. Right before her period, she took a blood test that showed her estrogen level was still a little high. The real news was that her FSH level was down to what could be considered a normal level—without drugs.

She got her period two days later, and it was a wonderful period—just like the old days. She started to feel a little hot during the day, but nothing like the hot flashes she had been experiencing. Her night sweats were also greatly reduced. The next month, Rita ovulated again—and this time an ultrasound showed that she was actually developing a follicle.

We continued acupuncture treatment on a weekly basis. Rita was able to ovulate three times. And on that last time . . .

I took a pregnancy test—and it came back positive! Dao told me I needed a blood test to make sure. That was positive, too. It was the shock of both our lives. We decided, for the first three months, to keep the treatment going to keep the embryo implanted. As far as I was concerned, whatever he said was gold at that point.

Throughout her pregnancy, Rita exhibited no pregnancy sickness. She was tired and had some asthma intermittently, but otherwise it was a symptom-free pregnancy with minimal complications.

It was a wonderful pregnancy. I think it shocked Dr. Dao, how powerful he was. I remember once asking him about the needles and how they worked. He said it was his energy going into the needles. I certainly felt that.

Before I had my daughter, I felt such a void. Something was missing, and I couldn't stop fighting to get it. I was relentless because in my heart I knew I was going to get it. And then she came to me, just as I knew she would.

In Rita's case, I think what made things work out was her extreme sensitivity—that and the fact that she was only thirty years old. If she had been thirty-five, I don't think we would have been able to achieve such success. She had such a strong reaction to acupuncture that her system allowed her to ovulate. And yet, when her doctor performed a cesarean section to deliver her daughter, he was dumbfounded because he could not find any ovarian tissue. A miracle.

12

PELVIC AND TUBAL

My husband and I tried to get pregnant for years. We started when I was about twenty-seven—I'm forty now. We stopped using birth control, and nothing happened. I went to my ob-gyn. We tried Clomid, insemination . . . nothing was happening. Only later on did we learn there was a problem with my tubes.—Mary

Tubal and pelvic diseases are among the most common infertility problems. They are probably the primary issue in about 30 to 35 percent of couples facing infertility.

The diseases of the fallopian tubes and pelvis can be traced to a number of different causes. For example, a woman with a history of infection might develop pelvic inflammatory disease (PID). Another example would be a woman with an anatomical abnormality—simply put, she was born with abnormal fallopian tubes. Yet another cause could be a blockage in the tube that prevents the sperm from reaching and fertilizing the egg.

The mechanism of the fallopian tube is very important. It needs to be free flowing; any obstruction or infection can create problems. Infections can damage the hairlike projections inside the tubes that are crucial for transporting the egg and the sperm. The way we frequently assess tubal blockages is to look at a woman's history of infections as well as whether there is a history of endometriosis. Often we will do a hysterosalpingography (see page 119) to see if the tubes are clear. If there are blockages or diseases in the tubes, usually an IVF procedure will have to be done in order to bypass the tubal blockage. Natural therapies have yet to prove strong enough to resolve most tubal blockage problems.

To give you one example: I had a patient who had scars that blocked both tubes. She tried IVF, using her own egg. It didn't work. So she moved on to donor egg.

DONOR EGG

When a patient's ovaries are compromised due to aging, disease, or other circumstances, sometimes a younger woman is sought to provide healthy eggs. After stimulating the donor's ovaries with drugs, the fertility specialist retrieves the eggs she produces. He or she then fertilizes these eggs with the sperm of the patient's partner and transfers them into the patient's uterus.

The transfer didn't work. I was puzzled—bypassing her tubes should have worked. To understand why it didn't, I went back to my notes on her case. I concluded that her tubes were creating problems because they were inflamed. They were sending pus down to the uterus and creating interference for implantation. I recommended that she have both tubes removed. She went back to the doctor who knew her case very well. He hesitated a little until he consulted with me. I told him that it needed to be done, that there was no advantage to leaving the tubes in there. He took them out, and the first transfer after that was a complete success. My patient got pregnant.

There are doctors who perform tubal surgeries as a way to clear tubal blockages, but the success rate of such surgeries to date has not been high because the more surgery is performed on the tubes, the greater the potential for additional scarring and even complete blockage of these delicate structures. In Chinese medicine, there are some reports that acupuncture and herbs have been successful in opening up tubes. Yet even here, the success rate has been low, falling somewhere between 10 percent and 30 percent.

Mary's Story

I first met Mary in February 1998, when she was thirty-two years old. For someone so young, she had a surprising number of health issues. She wanted to get pregnant but was realistic about her less-than-perfect health.

The things she had tried to improve her general health to that point hadn't worked. She knew she had to be in better shape before conceiving and was ready to work hard to achieve her goal of becoming a mother.

I had had acupuncture years earlier because I suffered from headaches. I liked it—as I far as I recall, it worked pretty well. But I didn't think about using acupuncture again until a friend of mine was diagnosed with Hodgkin's disease and started going to see Dr. Dao's brother to help her through the chemotherapy. I learned that Dr. Dao worked a lot with women who were trying to get pregnant. So I went to him, thinking he might be able to open my tubes using acupuncture.

Mary wasn't aware of it then, but a hysterosalpingogram would later reveal that her left tube was blocked and that her right tube was swollen like a balloon. The technical term for this swelling is hydrosalpinx. Because of this condition, Mary was carrying a lot of excess fluid in her body. But that was not her only problem. She suffered from lower back pain and frequent headaches that became more severe around the time of her period. She had very irregular cycles that ranged from thirty-two to fifty-two days. On top of all this, she had endometriosis, which caused her to have a heavy flow as well as clotting and cramping during her period. But what concerned me almost as much was her lifestyle. Mary had a demanding job that frequently left her overstressed and overwhelmed. Although she was diligent—perhaps because she was so diligent—her life was a lot to handle.

I wasn't stressed out or harried. I actually deal with stress very well. I do have a busy corporate job and commute a lot. My problem was that I wasn't in the best of health when I went to see Dr. Dao. Just before I did, I had a physical. My blood pressure and cholesterol were both really high. I remember they wanted to put me on high blood pressure medicine. I thought it was ridiculous— I was in my thirties.

Mary was an extremely smart woman with a very demanding life. Even though she had a positive outlook, you could just see the underlying anguish and sadness. Her problems with infertility had a strong effect on her. My goal was not only to regulate her body but to elevate her spirit by addressing her stress level, her lifestyle, and her diet.

Mary was somewhat overweight and was addicted to sugar. On that first day when I examined her, her pulse was thready, which indicated she might have low blood sugar (as it turned out, this was indeed the case). Her pulse was also rapid—a sign of a stressful life and perhaps inflammatory activity in her body. The tip of her tongue showed redness, which is usually the sign of someone with an overly active mind given to little sleep.

The first thing I did was ask her to cut out all sweets and alcohol.

I was open-minded. At that point, I really wanted to get pregnant. So I started seeing Dao weekly and started changing my whole way of living. I was overweight and felt crabby because I wasn't getting pregnant and because of the medications I was taking. I stopped eating sugar and started taking herbs.

We worked diligently to improve Mary's health. I began an acupuncture program to help regulate her ovulation and to address her other symptoms. Needles were inserted in her pelvic area, neck, and shoulders, as well as in her lower back and in certain areas of her arms and legs. I also prescribed a comprehensive formula of twelve herbs: angelica root, paeonia alba, ligustici, shisandia fruit, goji fruit, raspberry fruit, poria cocos, ginger, licorice, bupleuir, mint, and hawthorne berries. She responded very well to the treatments. Her energy became more stable and her body was in better overall shape.

By December of that year, we finally achieved a twenty-seven-day cycle with a normal flow and minimal clotting and cramps. Mary's stress didn't go away, but she was better able to deal with it. Her headaches and the tension in her neck and shoulders decreased. It was at this point that her fertility doctor and I asked her to have the hysterosalpingogram that revealed her tubal challenge.

At one point, Dr. Dao thought he could open the tubes through acupuncture. By this time, I had been going to him for several months and felt pretty great because of the treatments and the changes I had made in my lifestyle. But then he basically sat me down and told me that I needed to try something more serious, like IVF. It wasn't an either/or choice. He could still be helpful and instrumental during the IVF process.

With one tube blocked and the other swollen, it was unlikely that the sperm could ever swim through the tube to meet the egg. IVF would bypass her tube. In February 2000, she embarked on her first IVF. She responded decently to the drug stimulation of her ovaries, developing many follicles to spare. Unfortunately, Mary did not get pregnant. Her physician believed that the hydrosalpinx in the right tube was interfering with implantation in the uterus and advised her to have the right tube removed.

I had the surgery and then did another IVF. I still didn't get pregnant. I was clinging to this hope that it would all work out, and then . . . nothing. It was hideous. I put all my hopes on this one tube. When the IVF failed, I was crushed.

While Mary was going through her surgery and the IVF, I continued to support her body, using acupuncture and herbs to try to open her left tube. Even though it appeared to be open, I wasn't certain if this was just a temporary situation.

When Mary did the second IVF in July, everything looked good. She produced many follicles, of which sixteen actually fertilized. Four embryos of very high quality were transferred. She did get pregnant for a very short time but ultimately miscarried. It was devastating for her.

It took a few weeks before I was ready to go back to Dr. Dao. I remember he put a needle in my left lower leg and I screamed. The pain was incredible and so surprising because I never had felt pain from the acupuncture needles before. Dr. Dao explained the pain meant that I was ovulating on my right side. How strange was that? The side where my tube used to be? The side where my tube wasn't anymore?

In effect, Mary had just one right ovary and one left tube. In strictly scientific terms, the likelihood of getting pregnant in a situation like this is zero. Think about it for a moment: if you ovulate on the right ovary and you do not have the right tube, the egg is not going to get to the uterus and the sperm is not going to get to the ovary. But in Mary's case, the left tube must have "swung" over to pick up the egg—a very rare phenomenon indeed!

Guess what? After two IVFs and tubal surgery, I got pregnant naturally. My husband and I had gone on holiday. I don't know why I thought I was pregnant, but there it was. I remember seeing the little formation on the ultrasound on my birthday. My ob-gyn couldn't believe it. But Dr. Dao knew all along I was going to get pregnant. He told me so. Did the IVF jump-start things? I'm not sure, but I do think the acupuncture had everything to do with it. My little baby was meant to be.

I learned so much from Mary's case. Our ability to keep her left tube open and reduce the inflammation is probably the main reason why she could get pregnant naturally. Without a doubt, tubal problems take time to resolve. Even though an IVF procedure is still the ideal route to overcoming this challenge, it is not an absolute solution for mild to moderate tubal issues. Mary had other issues that needed to be addressed—and in a specifically holistic way. Putting her on an anti-inflammatory diet consisting of lots of leafy greens and virtually no refined sugar, caffeine, alcohol, or wheat is what really made a difference—that and her willingness to work hard and maintain a positive attitude, even when things were at their most bleak. I could not have done this without her help. We did it together.

Eastern and Western medicine are not exclusionary. Eastern medicine has been around for thousands of years. If you marry that knowledge to technology, it's brilliant. But you have to have persistence, and you have to have good support. I was lucky; my husband was always there for me. And my Western doctors had respect for Dr. Dao's methods.

How can I describe it? Dr. Dao is part physician, part psychologist. But you are the one who has to work on your own soul.

UTERINE

I knew I potentially had fibroids. I had the ultrasounds so that Dao was able to know what he was dealing with. I also knew we were both dealing with my age. And then there were the unknown questions.—Lori

The uterus is what we call the house of the fetus in Chinese medicine. It's the organ that helps carry the baby. Because of this great task, it needs to be both healthy and strong. The blood flow to the uterus must also be strong in order to create a thick and receptive uterine lining where the embryo can thrive. In a normal situation, the uterus is not an organ that becomes sick or diseased easily. Even when it does, it is still able to carry out a pregnancy quite well—at least, in most situations. Such is the power of the uterus.

Yet there are times when the uterus can present a challenge to a woman's fertility. One of them is a purely mechanical situation in which a benign growth, such as a fibroid or polyp, appears on the uterus. In another case, a woman can actually be born with an irregularly shaped uterus or one that is adhered (meaning the skin has folded over on itself). If the uterus is not in perfect working order, it can mechanically inhibit implantation by the fertilized egg. If a woman with a uterine abnormality does get pregnant, it can lessen her chances of carrying the baby to term.

If a woman has deficient levels of progesterone, weak egg quality, or weak ovulation, the sustaining nature of the uterus might be diminished. Sometimes we call this a poor or thin lining or an underdeveloped endometrium.

The only way to pinpoint the problem is to examine the condition of the uterus. We do this by using one or more of three basic tests. The first is the *hysterosalpingogram,* in which the doctor injects dye through your cervix, into your uterus, and through your fallopian tubes to allow a clear look at the shape of your uterus and the openness of the tubes. The second test is the *sonohysterogram,* which employs saline solution to bloat the uterus for better imaging. The third evaluation method is the *hysteroscopy,* in which the doctor sends a little camera through the cervix and into the uterus to see if there are any visible problems.

As I mentioned, the uterus does not become diseased easily, but when it does, it presents a special challenge. It is extremely difficult to treat a woman with large uterine fibroids while she is in the process of trying to get pregnant, because uterine fibroids are often fed by estrogen and tend to grow faster as pregnancy progresses. This is particularly problematic when a woman takes gonadotropins—medications that stimulate the ovaries to produce multiple follicles as part of IVF or stimulated insemination procedures. But even without stimulating drugs, fibroids can grow until they pose a threat to pregnancy.

Lori's Story

When I think of Lori, I am still amazed at how strongly her body wanted to be pregnant. And with so much working against her in terms of her fertility health, it appeared that the journey would not be an easy one.

Did I always want children? Oh, yes. I couldn't imagine children not being a part of my life. But after an early marriage at twenty-one that didn't last, I developed my own life and career. I was the marketing director for a couple of companies, traveled a lot, and then finally started my own company abroad. The years passed. And then one day, I decided it was time to come home to the West Coast. That decision came in part because I was reaching that age when I was thinking more and more about having children.

Then I met someone ten years my junior. The gods conspired, I guess. I was thirty-nine when we got married. Fairly soon afterwards, we started trying to have a baby. We tried without any intervention for eight months, to no effect. Every month that went by only made me that much more aware of how much time was passing.

Lori was forty-one when she visited me. Age was definitely an issue in her case. But there were other fertility challenges as well. She had been pregnant once, years earlier, but had spontaneously aborted at four weeks. Lori also had a history of fluctuating periods, starting as early as her teen years. Her periods were strongly irregular for nearly ten years before they stabilized. As she had gotten older, however, her period had once again begun to fluctuate. At the time I saw her, her cycle ranged anywhere from twenty-six to thirty-two days. She suffered pain—especially headaches—and dizziness during her period, along with clotting and a heavy flow. She also experienced lower back pain as a result of scoliosis.

I had practiced yoga for twelve years. I ran; I ate well; I tried to take natural herbs. I was very self-aware and understood my body intimately in terms of my cycle. I had gotten pregnant once, even though I miscarried. My gynecologist said there was no reason not to be pregnant.

Besides her history of menstrual irregularities, Lori showed signs of fibroids. In fact, three could be clearly visualized. They were all extending and protruding inside of her uterus. What's more, these fibroids were not small. Their presence completely distorted the uterine lining—what we call the endometrium. Positioned as they were, they created a potential challenge to the implantation of a fertilized egg.

As if this complication was not enough, Lori had had cervical surgery years ago after a pap smear revealed abnormal cells. Cervical freezing, known as cryosurgery or cryotherapy, is a common procedure for removing these abnormal cells. This entails applying liquid nitrogen at a temperature of approximately -50 degrees Celsius—in effect, freezing off the cells. Some normal cells are also damaged in the process, but most of the time they are replaced by new cells. The problem is that this can potentially alter the consistency of the secretion of cervical mucus and can compromise fertility potential. So Lori had many potential complications! And yet . . .

I wouldn't go through IVF. I did wait to have children because I wanted a partner, the right partner, for my child. If I couldn't do it naturally, it couldn't be right for me. The changes to my body, the rounds of expense—I knew the cycle of hormone therapy. I am still not convinced that we won't find out one day that there are deep medical repercussions to IVF. And so, based on what I knew, I wanted to stay holistic.

Dr. Dao understood that. I liked him a lot from the very beginning. I felt like an angel was surrounding me. I understood everything he explained to me about my condition. Unlike with other doctors, we had no communication problems. There's a strong spiritual element to what he does. Maybe that's why he came across as so sensitive. He had an ease in translating Chinese and Western approaches. I was ready to start working with him.

The first thing I discovered upon examining Lori was that her pulse was quite thin—a sign that her vitality level was low and that her reproductive essences were weakening. In addition, her tongue was quite pale, which suggested that her circulatory activity was a bit off and probably weak in the area surrounding her ovaries. Her tongue was also a little greasy, indicating that she most likely had a poor diet containing a lot of sweets. When she admitted to frequent bloating and problems with digestion, I knew we were on the right track. We talked about putting her on a program of herbal teas and weekly acupuncture treatments, and she readily agreed. I focused her acupuncture treatments on major points such as ST40 on her outer leg to help reduce her fibroids; ST28 and ST29 on the pelvic region to improve her ovarian functions; and SP6 on her inner leg near her ankle to regulate her endocrine functions and ovulation.

I also prescribed an herbal formula composed of cinnamon bark, dry ginger, Chinese angelica root, Chinese foxglove root, Asiatic cornelian cherry, cyberi herb, and Chinese yam for her specific conditions. The herbal ingredients combined to help strengthen her ovarian reserve, improve her digestion, and enhance her ovulatory regularity.

By the next week, Lori had gotten her period. According to Lori, there were already some changes. For one, her menstrual flow was lighter. There were fewer clots, and the color of the blood was much brighter. Her lower back pain and her excessive uterine contractions during menstruation had also improved dramatically. What's more, she wasn't experiencing the dizziness and headaches that so often accompanied her periods in the past.

I followed Dao's advice right from the start. But I was lucky—my obstetrician knew who Dao was and was open to my working with him. It's important for women to understand that not every obstetrician is as open to their patients being treated by a doctor of Chinese medicine. That openness is a key. It encourages you to follow Dao's treatment more rigidly. Within two months, I got pregnant.

We were suspicious of whether Lori was pregnant when she started to exhibit some unusual nipple sensitivity. The blood test confirmed it—she was pregnant. Unfortunately, the pregnancy was very, very weak. She lost the baby a few weeks later.

Lori's next period was very tough for her, both physically and emotionally. The bleeding was heavy and the cramps were so strong that they lasted for three weeks. The headaches came back; so did her lower back pain. All of the symptoms we set out to get rid of returned with a vengeance after her pregnancy failed.

At this point, we had to stop and take another look at all the factors in play. When Lori first consulted me, we identified that she had a uterine factor, a potential cervical factor, and an age factor. Now we had to add one more: a potential recurrent miscarriage factor. In addition, because of this quick pregnancy that did not sustain itself, the fibroids had grown at a rapid rate. It seemed the odds were really stacking up against her. Yet Lori was determined not to give up. From observing her physical reaction to her pregnancy—notably, her bloating and exhaustion—I realized that, before anything else, her fibroids needed to be tamed. I revised Lori's herbal formula and changed the selection of her acupuncture points to concentrate on shrinking her fibroids and improving her digestion. The herbal formula was composed mainly of daikon radish seed, perilla leaf, brassica seed, fritillaria fruit, citrus peel, mongolia bark, polygonus root, and hawthorne berry.

After the miscarriage, I kept trying to get pregnant. Dao had to change my herbal tea formula to keep the fibroids down; for my part, I was doing over-the-counter tests and keeping track of when I was ovulating. Everyone knew we were trying to have a baby and were very vocal with their opinions. By now I had been trying to have a baby for close to a year. It was frustrating—and stressful—but I knew she or he would come.

For the two months following her miscarriage, I continued to focus on shrinking Lori's fibroids and trying to get her body back in balance. Slowly, the herbal tea and acupuncture treatments began to have a positive effect on her system. Although her menstrual flow was still very dark, she started to feel less bloating and fatigue. Her period once again became more regular—this time coming at twenty-eight days. Unfortunately, she continued to have some nausea and a general sense of fatigue with her period. Once again, I adjusted her herbal formula by adding cyperi herb and astragali root, and changed the acupuncture treatment to assist her digestion and circulation. But the primary focus was still her fibroids. By her next period, the cramps were gone. There were very few clots and the flow was much, much lighter. She had better energy, too. And then . . .

Four months after my miscarriage, I got pregnant again. I have been clairvoyant for years. I understood—then and now—that this child was destined to be. I understood that, even though, as it turned out, my pregnancy was very hard.

Right from the start of her pregnancy, we closely monitored Lori's progesterone level. There are several things progesterone does to support a pregnancy. For one thing, it continues to ensure a good blood supply to the uterus, which in turn helps in the development of the placenta. Progesterone serves another important purpose. Since the fetus is like a foreign body to the mother's body, progesterone appears to decrease the maternal immune response to allow for the body's acceptance of the pregnancy. Finally, progesterone decreases the contractibility of the uterus. This helps to increase implantation. But despite the fact that Lori's beta numbers were rising strongly, her progesterone was not. We immediately made changes to her herbal tea to try to support her pregnancy and strengthen her progesterone. By the sixth week, her levels were much stronger.

Unfortunately, Lori's pregnancy symptoms became quite uncomfortable. She had headaches, bloating, and extreme nausea. Even more worrisome was the continued growth of her fibroids. By the eighth week of her pregnancy, I made the decision to focus on her digestive issues in order to

---

WHAT ARE BETA NUMBERS?

When you are pregnant, your body produces a hormone called beta human chorionic gonadotropin (beta HCG). Most of the time, this hormone is produced by the implanting embryo and can be detected as soon as eight days after ovulation. The beta HCG level rises exponentially during the first few weeks of pregnancy and reaches a peak level at about eight to ten weeks. It declines after that. Frequent blood tests to check for the appropriate rise of this number in the early part of pregnancy are done to ensure the viability of the pregnancy.

---

try to calm her stomach down. With the new treatment, she began feeling better—she still had some nausea, heartburn, and back pain, but nothing like before. The fibroids, however, remained a serious concern, despite our continued efforts to shrink them.

By the twenty-seventh week of her pregnancy, Lori's digestive system took a turn for the worse. An ultrasound showed that her fibroids had gone through a degeneration process, causing her severe pain. Once again, we modified the acupuncture treatments, this time to try and address the pain as well as the fibroids that caused them. By the thirty-first week of her pregnancy, Lori had developed toxemia, also known as preeclampsia. Toxemia is induced hypertension and is quite common in pregnancy. Mild toxemia usually does not pose problems for the mother and the child. But severe toxemia can cause many health problems for both. There is no known cause, but older women have increased odds of developing this condition.

After I found out I had toxemia, Dr. Dao and his herbs kept me out of the hospital. My blood pressure came down, and I was able to stay home. But then, at thirty-one weeks, I had what is called HELLP syndrome (hemolysis, elevated liver enzyme levels and a low platelet count). A very small percentage of women ever get it. I was hospitalized. . . . They didn't think I was going to make it. But my baby was born at thirty-two weeks. She weighed in at four pounds. And she was beautiful.

Honestly—and I believe this from the heart—the other doctors saved my life. But Dr. Dao helped me have my baby. I am a firm believer in my path and what the universe holds for me. All I know is that Dr. Dao is a miracle worker.

As I said, Lori's was an amazing journey—amazing because of all the challenges she faced; even more amazing because of her resilience. There's no other way to say it—Lori just had a strong spirit. She knew her body, she knew her limitations, and yet her strong spirit kept her going, no matter what life threw at her. From fibroids, to pain and loss, to toxemia, it kept her pushing onward to reach her dream. Hers is a spirit I will never forget.

CERVICAL

It's funny, but I had actually gone to Dr. Dao's clinic, the Tao of Wellness, a few years earlier. A friend had told me about this place that did acupuncture and Chinese medicine, so I went. I didn't see Dao, though; I saw someone else. She gave me herbs and acupuncture, and when I walked away, I thought it was all a crock—all these rich people with money to throw into alternative therapies. It just didn't work—that was my attitude then. But this time was different. I had a baby, and I lost him. This time, I wanted to make it a spiritual process. I wanted pregnancy to come naturally. In retrospect—and in my grieving—I thought it was wrong to do the drugs. It never crossed my mind that I would not be able to carry a baby.

Of course, I needed acupuncture—I needed a connection to my heart. That's why, before all this happened, Western medicine was better for me. I didn't have to access the rest of myself. But here it was. Life came knocking and asked: Are you ready? Because there's a whole new world for you to see.—Anna

One of the most important aspects of the cervical challenge relates to the cervical mucus, which plays several key roles in the reproductive process. For one thing, it takes on the ejaculated sperm in the cervix area and filters out abnormal sperm and debris. It also contains many nutrients that help nurture the sperm that do survive this selection process. You could say this mucus is really a kind of bank or reservoir for the healthy sperm. And when the sperm is in the presence of good mucus, it can potentially survive for longer periods of time. The mucus protects the sperm from aging and dying prematurely. In fact, I believe that the mucus actually makes the sperm even more active and alive.

But what if the mucus is less than perfect? Frequently when infections such as chlamydia, ureaplasma, or mycoplasma have occurred in the vaginal or lower intestinal tract, the result is a change in the consistency of the cervical discharge. That change, in turn, can weaken and even destroy the protective or nourishing characteristics of the cervical mucus. Aside from past or present infections, there is another factor that can affect the quality of the cervical mucus. When your hormone levels—particularly estrogen—are low, it can cause the mucus to be dryer and less functional.

Besides the mucus issue, the cervix itself acts as a gate that both protects and holds the pregnancy. In rare cases, the cervix can be closed, not allowing sperm to properly swim through it to access the fallopian tubes, where conception can occur. In other cases, the cervix is weak and can create potential problems during pregnancy by opening prematurely. In this case, a patient usually undergoes a procedure called cerclage, which involves temporarily sewing the cervix closed. A weak cervix during pregnancy is a frightening experience requiring a lot of bed rest and medical supervision. That was the case with Anna.

Anna's Story

I'm thirty-seven now, but I've wanted to have a baby from the time I got married. I was twenty-two then—I guess you could say I'm an old soul. I've always been ready for a child and figured, oh well, it'll happen. Then my dad got sick, and suddenly, I wanted to have a child right away. But nothing happened. My dad ultimately died, and I went through a grieving period. It was a while before I finally went to a doctor to deal with the fact that I wasn't able to conceive. She did a test and found that I had polyps in the lining of my uterus. It was the first I'd heard of it. I was willing to have them taken out, and I had the surgery.

When you are young, you are supposed to have fewer problems with infertility compared to older women. So clinically speaking, when a younger woman shows up in my office, I automatically anticipate that a greater challenge is at hand. In April 2001, Anna walked into my office for the first time. She told me the story of her difficulties in pursuing her dream of pregnancy. She was thirty-one years old and had been trying for more than eight years.

After the surgery, we kept trying—and trying. I bought ovulation kits, did the right things, but nothing happened. Eventually my doctor suggested we try Clomid. We did it for three rounds—and nothing happened. Our insurance wasn't covering things, and I was getting increasingly disillusioned. It's amazing how your life becomes so focused when you're trying so hard to have a child. I didn't see anything going on in my life clearly—my job, my marriage. It was profoundly disquieting.

My doctor finally saw that it wasn't working and said we needed to try the pros. At the same time, a very dear friend was going through IVF. Even though it was an extremely bad experience for her, they ultimately had their baby. My husband and I became godparents to their little girl. When we held her in our arms, something happened. We decided to go to the same fertility clinic my friend had used.

At the clinic, they said they didn't care what we had done before. As far as they were concerned, we were starting from square one. I told them that I had taken Clomid and that it hadn't worked, but they wanted to try it again.

WHAT IS CLOMID?

Clomid (clomiphene citrate) is frequently the first fertility drug used to stimulate the ovary. It is taken orally instead of by injection and is much less expensive than most fertility drugs. It is a potent drug and not without some side effects for some people. These side effects—besides multiple pregnancies—can include ovarian enlargement, hot flashes, pelvic discomfort, abdominal distention or bloating, nausea, vomiting, breast discomfort, eye or visual symptoms, headache, and abnormal bleeding. Clomid stimulates the body to produce more follicles. With this, hopefully the body will have more chances to get pregnant.

They also insisted that my husband get a complete workup. It was the first time that anyone had really acknowledged that he could be a part of this problem we were having. Sure enough—it turned out there were some problems with his sperm. This, in year seven of trying! But still, they chose to treat me.

By then I had turned thirty, and a trillion of our friends were having babies. I kept saying, "Great news! That's wonderful!" What I really wanted to do was jump off the Golden Gate Bridge. Then they discovered more polyps. After another surgery, my fertility doctor thought I should move on to injections. If the drugs didn't work, I would be on the IVF track.

So I injected myself and created more eggs to increase the chances of the sperm . . . and we got pregnant. I couldn't believe it. I was so excited. For me, it was the end of the journey. We found a very nice ob-gyn. I remember telling her I should be considered high risk given all I had gone through. But she reassured me that the whole idea of reproductive medicine was to try and get you pregnant. Once you are, you're fine.

So we went home and went about our lives. At three months, we sent out a little mailing, telling people we were pregnant. It was the best time of our lives. And then, a few weeks shy of my fifth month, I started to feel a little off.

One day, I set out to run an errand, though I wasn't feeling well. There I was, driving down the freeway, feeling horrible. I was in labor and I didn't even know it. I got off the freeway. My water had broken. I hadn't realized it. I was in a fabric store, on a cell phone, trying to tell my husband something was terribly wrong. I got back in the truck and drove straight to the hospital.

Fortunately, my husband had called ahead, so they took me right away. The doctor told me it was too late; there was nothing I could do. . . .

Our baby was born and died at the same time.

Anna came to me at a very painful time in her life. She had finally gotten pregnant after many years of trying, and she had miscarried later than most—at four months. After the miscarriage, she had had a D&C, a procedure to clean out her uterus, and had been spotting ever since. So it was a very difficult day for her when we met for the first time. But even under these overwhelmingly sad circumstances, I found her to be an extremely sweet and pleasant young woman with a strong determination underneath all of her sadness.

Our grieving process was intense. Our doctor's recommendation was to name our son. And that was what we needed to do. Afterwards, all I wanted to do was to see Dr. Dao. I didn't care how long it took to see him. I just wanted the next available appointment. I went with my husband. Dao looked at me and basically told me I was a mess.

Her pulse was thin and wiry, which told me that her blood was deficient and her hormone level weak. At the same time, she was tense and, understandably, emotionally distraught. Her tongue coating was thin, greasy, and white. That indicated to me that her digestive system was not working very well and that she was not absorbing nutrients. It also signaled that there was some yeast congestion or infection in her system.

Upon examination and listening to her history, I found that Anna had never truly had a regular period. Her periods had always been delayed, with thirty-two-day cycles. She had a very long menstrual flow, accompanied by severe cramps and clotting. When you counted the spotting, her period could last up to two weeks out of a single month. In some ways, Anna was always either bleeding or spotting. She also had recurrent polyps, which are more commonly seen in older women. That, to me, was an indication of a weak uterine environment. She had fibroid growth in her uterus that created a uterine receptivity problem. Obviously, the contributing factor to her fertility problems—both getting and staying pregnant—could simply be all of the excessive bleeding and inflammatory activity in her uterus.

I concluded that this case involved three main challenges. The first one was a male subfertility challenge. Even though her husband's semen parameters were suboptimal, I found this condition was easily correctable. I advised Anna's husband to seek a course of acupuncture and herbal treatments, which he did.

The second challenge was ovulatory. Anna had exhibited irregular ovulatory cycles that needed to be regulated. The third challenge was the uterine challenge. The scenario of excessive bleeding and severe menstrual cramps combined with polyps and fibroids was complex but not unmanageable. My first goal was to improve Anna's physical and hormonal health.

Dao told me that his goal was to try and get me healthy. He also examined my husband. Dao looked at his tongue and saw yeast in the back. He said one word: "control." He told my husband that he had issues with control and that it was coming from his stomach. My husband was floored. Here was someone who could tell exactly who he was just by looking at his tongue. Dao gave my husband herbal pills to treat his stomach. The amazing part is that my husband was willing to take them. As it turned out, he was incredibly impressed by the herbs and the acupuncture. He later said he felt great physically and that he had an almost meditative experience when he had acupuncture treatments.

We had lost our boy at the end of February. I told my doctor what we were doing, that I didn't want any Western intervention. She said go for it, even though she didn't think it would do any good.

I wanted to see if I could regulate Anna's period. It seemed to me, based on what she told me, that she had a short luteal phase. She would ovulate somewhere around the twenty-fifth or twenty-sixth day of her cycle and get her period on the thirty-second day. Her luteal phase lasted only seven or eight days, indicating that the synchronicity of both estrogen and progesterone was out of balance. Besides regulating her ovulation timing, I wanted to see if I could decrease Anna's excessively heavy menstrual flow and persistent spotting.

My second goal was to decrease her severe menstrual cramps, which were lasting several days, to the point where she was debilitated and weakened every month. Cramps occur when there are inflammatory activities, excessively thick lining buildup, fibroids, or any other factors that might disturb the normal blood flow and buildup of the uterine lining. In Anna's case, she had all of these factors. She needed a strong intervention to address her uterine lining buildup.

I mapped out a treatment program of acupuncture and herbal therapy. In her acupuncture treatments, I selected the main points of LV3, SP4, SP8, ST28, ST25, LI11, and DU20 to soothe her nervous system, regulate her ovulatory function, and decrease her cramps, flow, and spotting. I also prescribed an herbal formula composed of angelica root, gardenia fruit, peony root, and others to decrease her cramps, decrease her flow and spotting, decrease her fibroids, prevent polyp growth, and yes, stimulate earlier ovulation.

Anna's period after starting treatment showed that we had made great progress. She had a much less heavy period with reduced cramping. Since this was her first period after the D&C, it was a naturally delayed fifty-day cycle. To ensure Anna's progress, we continued the treatments. On her second menstruation since coming to me as a patient, she achieved a thirty-one-day cycle with a seven-day menstruation—a dramatic change from her usual thirteen-day period.

Her clotting also decreased, as did her menstrual cramps. Instead of several days of debilitating cramps, her cramps were now very manageable and did not render her dysfunctional. She felt happier and her energy had greatly improved.

Dao also told me that he wanted to work on my libido. And did he ever—I tell my friends, you should go! He gave me herbs that were amazing.

Anna's next period was the best she had had by far. Then, in June, around the tenth day of her cycle, she started to feel a pinch in her left ovary. Later we found that she had ovulated on the sixteenth day—much earlier than in the past. This indicated to me that her endocrine system was back in balance.

Anna got pregnant.

We couldn't believe it. We tried for three months, and I got pregnant naturally. But right away, I was nervous.

There was one thing that concerned me. Anna started having some diarrhea after getting pregnant. Her pregnancy sickness symptoms were strong, causing severe nausea. That prompted me to change her herbs to more traditional ones to support her pregnancy. The herbs included a small amount of ginger, atractylodis, scutellaria, citrus peel, and perilla leaves.

Despite ongoing treatment, all of her pregnancy symptoms continued to increase. She had nausea, vomiting, diarrhea, lower back pain, and pelvic twinges. In reviewing Anna's history of miscarriage, we realized that cervical competency might also be a problem. With that in mind, I gave her specific herbs to strengthen her cervix and uterus.

I remember I was on holiday. We talked on the phone, and he told me he was sending me fresh tea right away. It was Fed-exed. My in-laws thought I was out of my mind, but I didn't care. I was convinced I got pregnant because of him.

In Anna's eighth week of pregnancy, her nausea was so severe that she wasn't able to drink the tea, so I changed it to a pill form that had similar types of herbs. She continued to develop very strong digestive and gastric difficulties. Because of her history, her doctor convinced her to undergo a cervical procedure called cerclage as a preventive measure to protect against the loss of her baby. She had the procedure at about fourteen weeks.

I went into the hospital on 9/11. The date will always stay with me. After the cerclage, my doctor told me to just be careful and do moderate bed rest. But then, when I went in for my post-op exam, my cervix was funneling. From then on, I had to be on strict bed rest. I had one shower a week, a potty by my bed. That was it.

Funneling is a situation where even with a closure, the cervix is opening. Obviously, Anna had to be bedridden from this point on. In addition, her fibroids were growing and she was experiencing very severe stomach upset.

Frightened by the thought of losing another baby, Anna decided to give the herb tea another try instead of continuing to take the less potent pills. As if the cervical problem were not enough, her fast-growing fibroids began to flare up, causing contractions and abdominal pain. Sometimes they were quite severe, and her discomfort was strong. So, around the seventeenth week, I added another herb to the mix to try to shrink and calm down the fibroids.

The funneling did not continue, but there was real anxiety and concern. I stayed flat on my back, so I couldn't continue to have acupuncture. I ended up talking to Dao on the phone every week. And every week, he would modify the herbs.

Somewhere around the twenty-third week, Anna developed a urinary tract infection (UTI). Taking an antibiotic did not seem to help her, and she was having side effects from the drug: dizziness and more abdominal cramps. The cramps were persistent. So I further changed the herbs to deal with both the fibroids and the UTI. Then her obstetrician found out the baby's head was resting directly on the cervix, putting a lot of pressure on the fibroid. Every week there was a new development. We had to modify Anna's herbal formulation on a weekly basis.

Dao gave herbs to keep me strong, to keep the baby strong . . . and to help me when they discovered I had fibroids. I guess you could say I'm the queen of little problems in the reproductive world. One week, Dao told me he was going to China and to get herbs from his junior partner. But there was some confusion, and she wouldn't change the herbs because of her respect for Dao's knowledge. So I called my Western doctor. He told me to take Advil, even though he had told me earlier not to take it at all. I called Dao's office back and got his brother, who was so calm. He changed the herbs. I wondered: Is this really going to work? But that was my transcendent moment with Chinese medicine. I drank the herb tea, and the pain was gone. Nothing in Western medicine could do that.

By twenty-five weeks, Anna's fibroids became calmer as her UTI got better. Then she developed constipation as a result of taking antibiotics for her UTI. Again, I changed her herbs. Her fibroids and her abdominal pain got better. Then at thirty-one weeks, she found out that her baby was breech—rear-down instead of head-down in the uterus, a much more difficult position for birth. I gave her the traditional moxa stick (see box, "Moxa," opposite) and instructed her to do the treatment nightly for forty minutes with the help of her husband.

By thirty-five-and-a-half weeks, the moxa treatment didn't seem to have worked. The problem was that Anna was bedridden; she couldn't exercise or move around, so the baby could not turn. I told her to be patient, even though her obstetrician had advised a cesarean section.

By week thirty-six, the baby's head turned downward to normal presentation. In March 2002, Anna vaginally delivered Helen, six pounds and ten ounces of a happy, healthy spirit.

I feel so blessed to have my daughter. She's four-and-a-half now. Looking back, I can honestly say that both my husband and I were inalterably changed by Dao and by this whole life experience.

MOXA

What is moxa? It's a treatment that has been used effectively in traditional Chinese medicine for thousands of years. It involves burning a moxa stick (usually made from rolling the herb ai ye or mugwort leaves into a cigarette shape) close to the skin to warm the energy in a given acupuncture point so that local blood circulation can be increased.

In infertility situations, moxa is frequently used for pelvic cramps, poor ovulation, poor uterine lining development, and vaginal dryness, among other things.

In pregnancy, it is used to help turn a breech baby back to its normal position. This technique involves burning the moxa stick over one of the acupuncture points located on the outside corner of the root of the nail of the little toe. As the burning stick is held close to the feet, its warming effect travels up the acupucture channel toward the baby, encouraging it to move. Once the baby moves, gravity takes over, so the baby's head naturally moves down toward the pelvis. The advantage of this treatment is that it is a completely noninvasive and safe way to assist the baby to find the proper positioning for birth.

In the span of almost one year of taking care of Anna, I appreciated the resolve and never-ending positive energy and faith with which she undertook this process. I am indebted to her for this life-enriching experience.

I wasn't ready to have a child at twenty-two. I needed to learn. Now that I am a parent, I'm connected to my heart. Having a child is very challenging and sometimes painful. But it's wonderful, too. It's a reminder of where I've been and where I am now.

15

AUTOIMMUNE

I was pretty sick when I met my future husband. We dated for a few years, got married in 1998. Then, after three years, we decided we wanted to have a baby. I always knew it was going to be difficult. Later on, I learned that a lot of people with autoimmune illnesses had problems and that their ovaries aged faster than other people's. But at the time, I knew I just wasn't healthy.—Grace

Immunological challenges can be associated with not being able to get pregnant as well as with recurrent miscarriages. For example, people who have certain autoimmune diseases such as lupus, antiphospholipid syndrome, rheumatoid arthritis, multiple sclerosis, myasthenia gravis, Grave's disease, and diabetes mellitus have been known to have decreased pregnancy rates and increased miscarriage rates.

In order to understand why autoimmune disorders can increase the risk of infertility and miscarriage, it helps to know what these diseases actually are. They are a group of chronic disorders that are caused when the body's immune system for some reason attacks its own systems. These illnesses can involve virtually every human organ and system including the endocrine and reproductive systems. Many autoimmune disorders occur during a woman's childbearing years.

Many of these diseases are identifiable through symptoms, blood tests, or other evaluations. It is imperative to manage these conditions before embarking on trying to get pregnant. For one thing, these disorders could make it difficult to become pregnant. For another, they could worsen during pregnancy, resulting in miscarriage and even a life-threatening situation for you. Every miscarriage increases the odds of more miscarriages. Therefore, if you have an autoimmune disease, it is of utmost importance to prepare your body and to be in the best state of health possible before trying to conceive.

Consider natural therapies like acupuncture and herbs combined with a nutritional program specifically tailored to reduce inflammatory activities. Adhere to a strict healthful lifestyle and healthy eating habits. You need to work with a good physician who can help you manage inflammatory symptoms with drugs if the natural therapies don't work. The use of cortisone, blood thinners, or intravenous immunoglobulin (IVIG) during pregnancy has been recommended for some of these conditions to temporarily decrease immunological reactions.

WHAT IS IVIG?

Intravenous immunoglobulin is a serum solution of special proteins called globulins containing antibodies normally present in adult human blood. Globulins provide immunity against disease. By infusing IVIG into a woman's bloodstream, we attempt to modulate her immune system so that it is downregulated so as not to attack a pregnancy. Good management of autoimmune disorder symptoms has been known to increase the odds of a viable pregnancy outcome.

Grace's Story

When I met Grace in early December 2002, she was thirty-one, a pleasant, soft-spoken lady who had been trying to get pregnant. During her first visit, we discussed trying to manage some of the immediate health issues she was experiencing. The most apparent problem was that she had been suffering from psoriatic arthritis for quite some time. This is a skin condition called psoriasis that also affects the joints, causing chronic pain and swelling.

I had psoriasis; it developed when I was about fourteen. By the time I went to college, it had developed into arthritis, which basically attacked my skin cells. My knees were filled with fluid; it was very painful. Now it's different; there are wonderful drugs for my condition that work really well. But in 1989, I had to take all kinds of drugs. I'd be on them for a month, get my knees drained. . . . I felt the pain in every joint, from the bottom of my toes to my shoulders.

Back then I wasn't so compliant. But I managed to get into the groove so I could go on and live my life. I traveled, went abroad, and met my future husband while at college. Wherever I went, I made sure I made contact with a good doctor. I met a lot of rheumatologists, some of the best. It was a waxing and waning kind of disease. I was pretty sick.

Grace was suffering greatly from pain in her knees, in one elbow, and in her hands and shoulders. This had been going on for a long time.

She also suffered from a delayed menstrual cycle. When she was younger, she had been taking birth-control pills.

I was on the pill for about five years. When I went off the pill, I didn't get my period. Nothing happened—not that it really surprised me, given my history of sickness. I had this feeling that I needed to see someone to get things going. When I went to my gynecologist, I found out that I didn't ovulate. I did a cycle of Clomid, but nothing happened.

Now I had to see an infertility doctor. By sheer chance, I ended up with a wonderful one. The first time my husband and I went to see her, she thought we were really young to be experiencing problems. But I knew it wasn't normal not to ovulate for five months. And when they tested my FSH level, it was much higher than it should have been for my age.

I did more Clomid a couple of times, insemination about five times . . . and nothing happened. After about a year and a half, we decided it was time to move on to IVF. Maybe the eggs just couldn't fertilize. At least this way my doctor could see what was going on.

By now my husband and I had been married almost five years. I think I told two close friends about what we were going through. But of course, everyone knows you're trying. My doctor told me it was important for me to stay calm, especially because of my immune problems. But I think I must have cried for two years straight. I knew that it would be difficult, seeing everyone with kids, going to all those baby showers and birthday parties. But not being able to get pregnant was truly the most devastating thing I'd ever been through— more devastating than my illness, more devastating than anything else I had ever experienced. It was the utter despair of not being able to control what was happening—or in my case, not happening. I was going to therapy, I was being compliant . . . why couldn't I get pregnant?

I had the IVF. They didn't tell me until afterwards that my eggs looked "very odd." To me, that meant only one thing: bad eggs. It was my worst nightmare coming true. I had thought about adoption, and even using a donor egg. But neither choice seemed right for me. I was beyond devastated, but still not ready to give up. That's when my doctor suggested I see someone who had a lot of experience treating women who were going through IVF. She gave me Dr. Dao's name.

I walked into his office and I started crying.

Grace's eyes told me right away of her suffering. My heart sank; I felt her sadness. It was obvious that she was tired, to say nothing of her emotional and physical pain. She was trying so hard to get pregnant and all the while her body was giving her so much trouble. She had a chronic cough; she was also suffering from a delayed menstrual cycle. When Grace was younger and had been on birth-control pills, her cycles had always been twenty-eight days. Now her period was sometimes delayed— coming at thirty-five days—and her ovulation was fluctuating or not happening at all. She also had been experiencing some very light spotting for eight days after she ovulated. This had been the case for three cycles before she came to see me.

I looked at Grace's tongue, and it appeared redder than it should have been—a sign of severe inflammatory activities in her body. Her pulse was wiry. This indicated to me that the chronic inflammation in her body was so great that the pain it created had begun to affect her entire being. The first thing I had to do was address her psoriasis and her arthritis.

I was very impressed, because Dr. Dao was extremely knowledgeable about rheumatoid arthritis and IVF. I found out he used to run an arthritic clinic in China. I thought I was going to an acupuncturist. I wasn't expecting so much medical knowledge.

Besides addressing her inflammation, I wanted to see if I could regulate Grace's hormones so that she could ovulate on time. I was concerned about her delayed periods. So together we mapped out our treatment plan. I suggested that we meet once a week for acupuncture.

I thought he was extremely happy and positive. That was important to me, especially since he urged me to try and keep an optimistic outlook. He told me it was especially important to keep my immune system calm. Otherwise, it would attack my ovaries and decrease my egg quality. The whole idea of his treatment was to get me ready for my next IVF cycle.

Unfortunately, when I saw Grace again, the pain in her knees was so severe that it almost inhibited her from walking.

I was still taking medicine for my arthritis—Enbrel. I was very, very sick.

I decided the acupuncture treatments should address her pain. I did this because pain can really interfere with the ability to get pregnant. I felt that was the case with Grace.

So we started a special treatment of acupuncture where we used very small microcurrent impulses sent through needles to reduce the pain. We worked on the knees aggressively yet gently, since these were the joints that bothered her the most. Each time after we did the treatment, she seemed to feel a little better. It gave her some temporary relief. At the same time, I also tried to strengthen her energy. She was still coughing a lot, and she was still having a lot of spotting after ovulation.

He must have made me ovulate really well. I don't even know why my husband and I tried that month—I was just waiting to get my period. I wasn't using any fertility medication at all. After just one month of treatment with Dao, I got pregnant.

At the time, it seemed like the pregnancy itself helped—at least in the beginning—to temporarily relieve Grace's arthritis. But because of her fear of the side effects and possible unknown adverse efffects of the arthritis medication on the health of her fetus, Grace decided to stop taking medications when she reached her sixth week of pregnancy.

I didn't take any medicine at all. I was so scared. I was basically in bed for the whole time. I was never sicker.

Without the medication, Grace's joint pain increased greatly, so during the first trimester, I continued with the electroacupuncture treatment to give her some relief from her knee pain. Unfortunately, she also suffered from pregnancy sickness, with a lot of queasiness, poor appetite, and vomiting, but by the time she was twelve weeks along, all of these pregnancy symptoms had gotten better.

Because of the severity and persistence of her joint pain, however, her doctor recommended that she take cortisone. She was on the medication for the rest of her pregnancy and was able to deliver a little girl.

My daughter is so delightful. But back then, after I had her, I had a postpartum flare-up of my condition and had to go back on powerful arthritis drugs. Because they were so toxic, I also had to go back on birth-control pills. But I thought of having another baby. This time, I didn't wait to see Dr. Dao. I knew it was he who had helped me get pregnant before.

Grace came back to see me in August 2004. She had been on birth-control pills, but she went off them around that time to try to get pregnant again. She still had her knee problems, with swelling and joint pain. But this time, she had an additional problem: her prolactin level was elevated. When this hormone becomes elevated during regular menstrual cycling, it is called hyperprolactinemia. This can be due to tumor growth in the pituitary, thyroid disease, or polycystic ovarian disease, among other factors. When the prolactin level is elevated, it reduces the production of two hormones necessary for ovulation: follicle-stimulating hormone (FSH) and gonadotropin-releasing hormone (GnRH). Both of these hormones are needed to grow your eggs and to help you ovulate—crucial when you are trying to get pregnant. Grace's doctor had prescribed medication to reduce her prolactin level, but it was still quite high. Fortunately, her ovarian reserve seemed to be intact and quite good. But her ovulation was irregular.

By looking at her tongue and taking her pulse, I realized that Grace's energy and strength had diminished a little since her first pregnancy. I made some modifications in her herbs to improve her vitality and give her more strength. Later I found out that her blood tests indicated she was borderline anemic.

In March 2005, her doctor prescribed a drug to induce ovulation. She got pregnant. Better still, her pregnancy seemed solid.

The first time around, I stopped seeing Dr. Dao after my first trimester. My child, though healthy, was born prematurely. I wanted to ensure that wouldn't happen again. I kept up the treatments with Dr. Dao pretty much throughout my second pregnancy.

We consulted a perinatologist, who recommended that Grace continue taking arthritis medication to minimize the risk of another premature delivery. It worked. She delivered her second child at thirty-eight weeks and six days.

The odds were so stacked against me. But I wasn't about to give up. Part of what helped me was Dr. Dao's relentless optimism. He told me he could make me have better egg quality, and he did. And he was just as honest about what he couldn't do in terms of my autoimmune problems. I so appreciated that.

I thought he was just like everyone else. He proved me wrong.

16

MISCARRIAGE

I got pregnant—again with twins—and followed my doctor's advice to the letter. I was on all kinds of estrogen, progesterone, and blood thinners . . . everything that was supposed to help me keep my babies. I was like a human pin cushion. And then, at twelve weeks, just when I was supposed to be out of the woods . . . the same thing. Ultrasound, and no heartbeats. I lay there on the table and just stared at the ultrasound monitor. I couldn't even breathe, let alone cry.—Paulette

What do we mean when we talk about recurrent pregnancy losses? Women who have had three or more miscarriages fall into this category.

There are many reasons for recurrent miscarriages. For example, they could be genetically related, stemming from an abnormally shaped uterus. In the 1950s a drug called DES (diethylstilbestrol) was prescribed to pregnant women—ironically enough—to prevent miscarriage. Some baby boomers were born with reproductive system abnormalities because their mothers took DES. When a uterus is not a normal shape, it cannot carry a child well. The result is that the fetus frequently grows to a certain number of weeks of gestation and then a miscarriage occurs because the placenta cannot develop well in a uterus not strong enough to support a pregnancy.

DES is not the only thing that causes abnormalities in the uterus. There are women who simply have a weak uterus because of poor health or poor blood circulation. In these cases, the uterus can't support a pregnancy. Parental chromosomal abnormalities cause recurrent miscarriage in roughly 5 percent of couples. When one or the other partner has a chromosomal abnormality, it increases the probability that the fetus will also have chromosomal imbalances or problems.

Then there is the aging issue. In fact, this seems to be the most frequent cause of miscarriage when all the other factors are ruled out. As a woman ages, her egg quality decreases. A less-than-healthy fertilized egg develops into an embryo with abnormal or unbalanced genetic material, which in turn can result in a miscarriage. An older woman might also have a weaker uterus; in addition, she is more likely to have uterine fibroids or polyps that inhibit implantation. If she has surgery to remove these fibroids or polyps, there is an increased chance of scar tissue or damage to some major arteries supplying blood to the reproductive organs. All of these situations decrease the potential for pregnancy.

We also know that miscarriage can occur because of immunological and autoimmune disorders. But there are many other factors as well, including forms of hidden cervical or vaginal infections such as chlamydia, toxoplasma, ureaplasma, mycoplasma, bacterial infections, herpes virus, and even cytomegalovirus infections.

Environmental factors such as smoking, the use of alcohol, and heavy coffee consumption can play a role. All have been known to create or predispose a woman to pregnancy loss. Endocrine factors such as low thyroid levels and unstable blood glucose are tied to miscarriage; so are problems with metabolism, diabetes, and low prolactin levels. In short, there are many different challenges that can cause miscarriages: genetic factors, anatomical factors, immunological factors, hemophilia, endocrine factors, environmental factors, and infectious states. And these are just the causes that we know about. Many times, even a thorough and systematic evaluation can't provide a clue as to why a woman miscarried. In my experience, these are the most difficult cases of all.

If you have had two or more miscarriages, it is extremely important to get a comprehensive evaluation before trying to get pregnant again.

Paulette's Story

I first met Paulette in October 1997. She was forty-one years old and had already experienced two miscarriages. She was not unlike many of the women I see at my clinic who come to me after suffering the loss of one or more pregnancies. Most of the time, there are no clear-cut reasons for these miscarriages, with the possible exception of advancing age. But Paulette's case was different. . . .

I married late. I didn't think I would have a difficult time getting pregnant, but I also knew from what I had read that my fertility wasn't exactly in full bloom at the age of thirty-eight. My husband had had a vasectomy, but then he had it successfully reversed. So there was this slight glitch going in, but we were pretty confident that we wouldn't have a big problem getting pregnant. At least that's what my gynecologist told me.

In her early thirties, Paulette was diagnosed with uterine fibroids, which she had surgically removed. Later on, it was revealed that she also had a septum in her uterus. Unfortunately, by this time, she had already had two miscarriages.

UTERINE SEPTUM

A uterine septum occurs when the uterus is not properly formed at birth. It can cause difficulties in both conception and pregnancy.

Your uterus began to form around the second or third month of your mother's pregnancy. The uterus is basically formed from two tubelike structures, called müllerian ducts, fusing their middle portions. The upper portions of these tubes develop into fallopian tubes. The fused midsection continues to grow, ultimately becoming the uterus. As the uterus enlarges, the area where the tubes touch each other dissolves, leaving one hollow uterine cavity.

There are times when things do not go as planned. When the ducts do not merge, a double uterus may form. When the ducts merge partially, this can create a heart-shaped (bicornuate) uterus. When one duct fails to develop, this can create a single-horned (unicornuate) uterus with only one fallopian tube. When the fused area of both ducts does not dissolve, this can create a dividing wall in the uterus otherwise known as a uterine septum.

> The septum varies in size and may or may not present a problem. The septum "hangs" from the top of the uterus and can reach down to the uterine opening. The larger the septum, the more likely it will interfere with conception and pregnancy. Frequently a physician can use ultrasound to assess whether a septum needs to be removed. An outpatient surgical procedure called a hysteroscopic resection can be performed to remove the septum. The success rate is high and the recovery is relatively fast.

After a few months of trying without success to conceive, my gynecologist suggested that I try artificial insemination. Even though my husband's vasectomy reversal was successful, there wasn't a whole lot of sperm to work with. There was some process where they spun the sperm to concentrate it, then did the insemination. I also had to take a drug, Clomid, which had a lot of side effects. It was supposed to ensure one or more good eggs, but it basically made me crazy. It was like the worst PMS I'd ever had. Anyway, my husband and I tried two or three rounds of insemination. When nothing happened, the doctor suggested I try the next step—a fertility doctor who specialized in IVF.

I ended up with a doctor who basically took one look at my age and decided that I needed a lot of drugs to help me produce eggs. I was still very naive at the time, even though I had read a lot about IVF and what it really entailed. I tried not to think about the amount of drugs I was injecting myself with, because I figured it was what I had to do to have a baby. I also thought I was in good hands. Instead, I ended up in the hospital with so many eggs inside me that it took hours to retrieve them. It took at least three months before my body was back to normal, or calm enough to accept the fertilized embryos made from my eggs and my husband's sperm. I remember one of the nurses telling me I could be an egg donor—she'd never seen anybody my age react to the drugs so strongly. Forget that I had almost died from being overstimulated.

But it all seemed worth it when I got pregnant with twins. Everything seemed okay, even though I was put on more drugs—progesterone and estrogen. I remember reading the label on the estrogen patch and seeing in big black print: "Do Not Use If Pregnant!" The doctor told me to ignore it, that the

rules didn't apply when you were doing IVF. It was like everything was back-
wards. But I did it.

    I miscarried right around the end of my first trimester. No warning—the
ultrasound couldn't pick up the heartbeats anymore. I was devastated. The
worst was the doctor's dismissive approach when I tried to find out why: I was
forty—what did I expect?

When Paulette first came to see me, I listened to her history. She was obviously very upset and anxious to know why she had miscarried. I explained how I would assess her, using the standard traditional Chinese medical approach. When I took her pulse, I found it wiry and thready. A wiry pulse is a tense pulse usually found in a body marked by pain or lacking in proper rest. And Paulette did, in fact, confirm that she had chronic back and pelvic pains. She also suffered from a long-term restless sleep condition. The thready or weak nature of her pulse is usually found in patients with poor circulation who are anemic or fatigued. This was the case with Paulette, who had been diagnosed with chronic fatigue.

Her tongue appeared to be slightly greasy, thin, and yellow, which indicated indigestion and a sluggish bowel movement. Her menstrual cycles were regular but delayed, about thirty-five days.

But what concerned me the most was her uterus, which had a signifi-cant history that couldn't be ignored. Aside from having uterine fibroids, she had had a septum removed in a recent surgical procedure. This indi-cated to me that her uterine receptivity was questionable and that her ability to sustain a pregnancy had been diminished.

In Chinese medicine, the uterus is considered the "house" for the fetus. It is an organ that is strong and has a rich blood supply. Like a house, its walls need to be strong, and the inside needs to be warm and habitable. In traditional Chinese medicine, many bodily systems and organs such as the endocrine system, the nervous system, the heart, and the liver have a direct connection to the uterus. Any changes in health status can affect the normal functioning of the uterus, especially in women with advancing maternal age. In Paulette's case, there were several challenges that had to be faced.

The thing that I remember most about my first visit with Dr. Dao is how
unrushed it all seemed. I had all this misery and sadness bottled up inside me,

and I needed to get it all out. So I kept talking faster and faster, aware of my watch, wondering how much I could tell him about what had happened to me before he told me my time was up. But he never did. He sat and listened to everything, and when I was all talked out, he started asking questions. All kinds of questions about how I felt physically, then how I felt emotionally. . . . It wasn't my typical doctor experience.

When the uterus is in trouble, it's usually because of one of three reasons. As I've mentioned, the first is the shape of the uterus—a genetic issue. A person can be born with an abnormally shaped uterus, sometimes with a septum growing inside. If the deformity is mild, a woman can still get pregnant. But if there is a septum long enough to begin to divide the inside of the uterus, surgical removal is usually required. The result is that the uterus may have difficulties holding multiple gestations at the same time, which is possibly why Paulette miscarried twice with twins.

The second threat to the uterus comes when there are fibroids. The uterus is a muscular organ. But sometimes, for unknown reasons, some of the areas of the muscle layers can begin to grow uncontrollably. Extra muscle nodules—called fibroids or myomas—appear. If these myomas are small and not immediately in the embryo's favorite area of implantation—the fundus—a woman can still conceive and can likely have a viable pregnancy.

The third threat to the uterus is infection or endometriosis. Infections can damage the inside wall of the "house." In the old days before the availability of penicillin, uterine infections were common. Today infection in the uterus is more rare and treatable. The usual symptoms are tenderness of the uterus, lower abdominal discomfort, offensive and profuse vaginal discharge, and slightly raised body temperature and pulse. The uterus may be infected by a variety of bacteria: the signs and symptoms vary according to the organism as well as the severity of the infection. Uterine infection can cause adhesions, where the uterine walls stick together. This is commonly called Asherman's syndrome. This condition can cause painful menstruation and may block blood from leaving the cervix.

The most common cause of Asherman's syndrome is the presence of some products of conception in the uterus. This can come from a small portion of the placenta that failed to be discharged in abortion, miscarriage, or a normal pregnancy delivery. Any foreign body left behind creates an ideal culture for bacteria—hence, infection. An ultrasound scan can assess whether there are any retained products of conception within the uterus. The treatment is usually a course of antibiotics with hysteroscopy if removal of the product is necessary. Sometimes a balloon is inserted and retained in the uterus for a short period of time to prevent further development of uterine wall adhesion.

Endometriosis, in contrast, is not unlike leaking pipes causing mold growth inside a wall of a house. Either way, the uterus can become uninhabitable.

In Paulette's situation, her house had had an extra wall (the septum) and nasty bulges (fibroids). Both had been cut out, but while the surgical procedures were meant to increase implantation of her embryos, there was also the possibility that they weakened the uterus and actually decreased the chances of conception and of holding onto the pregnancy. My priority was to find ways to heal and strengthen Paulette's uterus before she attempted another round of IVF.

I was eager to go ahead and try another IVF. I didn't want to wait for three months, which is how long Dr. Dao suggested we'd have to work together. I felt I was running out of time. I knew in my heart I would get pregnant again. But I was afraid of another miscarriage. So I figured I would try to follow what he told me to do.

Two of the best ways to strengthen Paulette's uterus were to increase the localized blood flow and the available nutrients. With that in mind, I customized an herbal formulation that would nourish her blood and improve her circulation. I also embarked on a weekly acupuncture treatment to guide and improve the blood flow to her uterus, and to improve her ovulation, which was sluggish and somewhat delayed. I chose acupuncture points ST36, SP6, Zigong, LI11, and DU20 as the base acupuncture formula in strengthening her blood flow and her vitality, and to improve her digestion and absorption.

I wasn't crazy about the herbs, especially since it took an hour to make them into a tea every two days. But I didn't mind the acupuncture treatments at all.

The needles weren't painful; I barely felt them. I just remember lying on the table in this darkened room, with a heat lamp over me, listening to some beautiful Chinese music. . . . Usually, I fell fast asleep.

Because of her sensitivity and overreaction to drugs—especially the fertility drugs used in her IVF procedures—Paulette reacted to the acupuncture and the herbal treatments in a positive manner. Her chronic lower back and pelvic pain decreased significantly during these few months of therapy, indicating that the blood flow to her pelvic cavity had improved greatly and that inflammatory activities in these regions had been reduced. At that point, I believed that her uterus would be able to carry a viable embryo to term. And because her prior IVFs had yielded many embryos that appeared to be of good quality, I felt she was still a good candidate for IVF—despite her age.

After another IVF, with five embryos transferred, Paulette got pregnant.

I was sure I'd get pregnant. But I was also sure another miscarriage would destroy me. I was a nervous wreck until I learned that I was carrying one baby this time, instead of two. Somehow I thought that would make things all right, that the pattern was broken. I basically held my breath for the first four months and continued to see Dr. Dao for treatment. I never felt sick; in fact, I never felt better. My baby boy was born full term, big and healthy. He was breech, so I had to have a C-section. Otherwise, everything was wonderful—so wonderful that it wasn't long before I decided I wanted to take one more try at having another baby. I remember talking to my fertility doctor about it, and he was very forthright about how I had managed to beat the odds. It's interesting, because most fertility clinics base their "success" figures on how many women manage to get pregnant using IVF. I didn't realize—or maybe I didn't want to—that most of those pregnancies didn't result in a baby.

Even so, I made up my mind to try another IVF. I figured I had one miracle; I was willing to try for another.

Knowing that Paulette would want to try to get pregnant again soon, I examined her a few weeks after her cesarean section. She appeared happy, tired, and anemic. The pregnancy had taken a toll on her body—

her lower back pain had returned. Having a child in your forties is not easy. It takes a lot of energy and it also weakens the blood. I changed my acupuncture points to SP3, SP6, ST41, CV4, CV6, and CV12 to better fortify her blood and to help her recover from her surgical delivery.

Eleven months after her cesarean section, Paulette embarked on another IVF.

The IVF worked beautifully. The doctors were pointing the embryos out like proud fathers. Lots of cells, just perfect. They implanted five. . . . Then it came time for the sonogram. Twins. My heart sank. I knew right then and there it wasn't going to work, and nothing the fertility doctor could say could reassure me. Dr. Dao also understood my concern, but he tried to keep me calm. I kept going for treatment with him and for my sonograms with the fertility doctors. One day, there it was . . . no heartbeats. Another miscarriage. I was beyond devastated. And yet not surprised.

The miscarriage was understandably difficult for Paulette. And yet at that point I knew that with her track record of four pregnancies and three miscarriages, she would most likely get pregnant again. But it was also increasingly apparent that her uterus had become the key issue in this situation.

I decided to change her herbal formula. I was also able to persuade her to wait for a few more months before she tried again with the frozen embryos left over from the previous IVF. In analyzing Paulette's past history and focusing on her weakness in the blood, I decided to add radix astragali and mulberry to her regular formula. These two herbs in combination enhance blood production and provide nourishment to the uterus and to the body in general. I was hoping this would help her to carry the pregnancy better.

Following a successful embryo transfer, she achieved a viable pregnancy and delivered at term.

In my heart, I knew I was going to have children. I wasn't sure how, and I wasn't sure how long it would take. It's what kept me going. Looking back on it now, I can see how fortunate I was to be able to do all of these high-tech procedures—many women can't afford them. Do I ever wish I hadn't waited so long to have children? Sometimes I think it would have been so much easier if I had started trying to have a family when I was younger. But that's not how it turned out. I'm just extremely grateful that it all worked out in the end.

Paulette learned about her deficiencies but had a plan—and she stuck to it. She was very persistent and faithful with her weekly acupuncture treatments and drank her herb teas regularly. It was not an easy journey. It was full of ups and downs: excitement, disappointment, sadness, and happiness. She held on, steadfast, and knew what she wanted. She was very fortunate—I'd have to say more fortunate than most. Against all odds, she was able to have two children.

17

CONSTITUTIONAL

Basically, I was born with a hole in my heart. I wasn't getting enough oxygen. When I was five, I had a correction. The doctors did a procedure that helped provide oxygenated blood. Afterwards, I functioned well, doing all the normal things. The doctors said at some point my heart would probably have to work harder than it had to, and that I may need to have my pulmonary valve replaced.

When I was five, they did a full open-heart surgery and patched the hole. It was considered a full correction of the problem. They weren't replacing the valve because I was still growing. This was back in the sixties. Now, of course, the technology is such that they could replace the valve right away, allowing a longer life span for the valve.

By the time I reached early adulthood, I basically forgot about it and went through life. Although I think my heart issue is part of what shaped me.—Julianna

Other fertility challenges mostly relate to a person's health state. There are times when we feel that a patient is not in the most suitable health to carry a child. I think it's very important to work closely with a patient who has such health issues, because the consequences of having a child when you are not healthy can be quite serious both for the mother and for her offspring.

As healers, we are also ethicists. We must practice our medicine in the most ethical manner. That's why we need to evaluate the patient's health and make suggestions about how to improve it, whether it means changing a work situation, lessening stress, or bolstering a weak constitution. By addressing these challenges, we can help a woman increase her fertility potential.

Julianna's Story

Julianna was thirty-six years old when she first came to my office. She is a wonderful woman, very sweet and very compliant with her treatments. Her history has been just amazing.

> *I got married at thirty-one. My husband and I started thinking about having children a few years after that. I guess you could say I was in no rush. Anyway, I had been going to a cardiologist on a regular basis because of my heart issues. When I started thinking about having children, I started talking to my cardiologist.*

Julianna had had another operation on her heart two years prior to seeing me. Listening to her story and reading her records, it was clear that she had gone through a lot of major surgeries and had serious issues regarding her heart and her blood flow.

> *The cardiologist was honest with me. What it basically came down to was this: If I wanted to have children, I should replace my heart valve sooner rather than later. Starting a family with my heart as it was might aggravate my condition. My feeling was to just do it and get it over with. That's how I came to have open-heart surgery at the age of thirty-four.*
>
> *After the heart surgery, I was told to wait for a year before trying to have a baby so that I could have a chance to get back to normal. They fixed my heart, all right, but it did take a toll. Eight or nine months later, I still didn't feel right. I had already had a bout with pain two years earlier when I had back surgery to repair some lower back disks. To control the pain, I started going to a Chinese acupuncturist instead of taking the steroids the doctors wanted to prescribe. I also started doing yoga.*
>
> *We started trying to have kids when I was thirty-five. My husband and I decided we would go to a certain point to try and get pregnant—and not go beyond it. I didn't want to take drugs or do IVF or anything else physical. I didn't want to put my body through more than it had already gone through. For me, it had to be natural. I didn't even want to take tests, as my ob-gyn suggested. I felt, why bother if I wasn't going to do anything about it? I figured, if*

there's something blocked, if there's something preventing pregnancy, then that's just the way it was. I couldn't make my body do something it couldn't.

We tried for a while, and it wasn't working. A friend of mine had gone to Dao after years of drugs and infertility treatments, and it worked for her. So we decided to give it a shot.

In our initial consultation, Julianna described frequent feelings of light-headedness. She had been experiencing irregular menstruation for more than one year, with her period fluctuating between twenty-three and twenty-eight days. She would spot excessively, both at the beginning and at the end of her period. All told, her periods would last a total of six days. Sometimes her flow was moderate; sometimes it was heavy. According to Julianna, her blood was usually bright red but without real clots. She also experienced some mild cramps.

The light-headedness was a real concern to me, especially when I learned that her energy had always been very unstable around the time of her fluctuating periods. This woman had had three chest surgeries and one back surgery. To me, her condition indicated that her blood flow was not good. Her pulse confirmed this. It was very, very feeble. By that I mean I could hardly feel it. I had to press as hard as I could to try and find a pulse. The pulse symbolizes the strength of the heart. And that strength—or lack of strength—had a lot to do with Julianna's weakened heart state and the difficult surgical procedures that she had endured.

Fortunately, her tongue exhibited a normal pink color. That indicated to me that even though she had undergone these heart procedures, there was still a sufficient blood flow to supply all her internal organ systems. So, in effect, she was not suffering from any kind of ill health. Yet her body was in a fragile and weak state. In talking with Julianna, I also discovered that she didn't sleep well. In fact, her sleep had always been shallow. Given her other factors, I knew we had to do something to improve her rest.

My first time seeing Dr. Dao was great. I thought to myself, why can't all doctors be like him? We talked a lot about the heart stuff. He felt that had he known me before, he could have helped get my immune system boosted and in better shape. I didn't disagree. It certainly would have been nice to gear up before the surgery and to have gone into it stronger.

You know, Chinese medicine is very much about helping yourself. Part of the problem with Western medicine is that it is so institutionalized. You get so accustomed to Western doctors who feel they fixed you. "You can go now, it's okay." Or, "Here's the problem, take this pill, this will do it." My heart surgery, my back surgery—I never really associated them with my body. But trying to have a baby was a much more emotional and mental thing for me. I felt if Dao's treatments could work, they would work because he was just helping my body do what it was meant to do.

At our first meeting, we also talked about tests that Julianna's husband had taken to determine the quality of his sperm. Even though the shape or form of his sperm could have used a little improvement, his sperm quality was good enough to be able to get her pregnant. The focus would be on Julianna.

I proceeded to give her acupuncture treatments, selecting points such as ST36 on her outer legs, LI10 on her forearms, LU9 on her wrists, and CV4 and CV6 on her pelvic midline. These points were all very good for strengthening Julianna's vitality, nourishing her blood, and facilitating her circulation. I also prescribed an herbal formula to address her condition. One of the main herbs I used was codonopsis root, a very versatile herb traditionally used to enhance vitality, improve blood production, and strengthen heart functions. The other herb was cuscuta seed, a common herb used in infertility conditions that is excellent for strengthening follicle quality and libido.

About two weeks after we started treatment with acupuncture and herbal teas, Julianna got her period. There were already some encouraging changes. The spotting during the first two days had become minimal; she menstruated for two days and then spotted only at the end. Her energy had improved, and she admitted she generally felt better. By the time she had her second period, her flow was considerably heavier. That was a very good sign, because it indicated that her body was producing more blood and that her uterine lining was getting thicker. Her energy continued to get stronger.

The main concern was that she still had considerable spotting at the end of her menstrual flow. This indicated to me that her estrogen and progesterone production was probably low; the spotting could also be connected to her heart issues. I intensified her herbal prescription to nourish her blood production and heart function. I added artemisia leaf and ligustri fruit to her formula to control the blood flow and eliminate the spotting. Ligustri fruit is also known to nourish and help hold the uterine lining. With these two synergistic combinations, we were able to reduce Julianna's spotting and improve her menstrual flow.

When the spotting began once again the following month, we thought her period might be starting again. Instead, she was pregnant.

It might have been as simple as a hormonal imbalance or circulation problems related to my heart. Or maybe it was that after being so run-down, I was more in balance. All I know is that within two months of treatment, I got pregnant. I went to Dr. Dao all through my pregnancy, once a week. I felt in tune with my body, that I was nurturing it.

At a little over six weeks, Julianna went in for an ultrasound and we saw a healthy fetal heartbeat. This was very encouraging, even though she was often fatigued—something I continued to address with herbs and acupuncture throughout the pregnancy. When she exhibited some mild nausea from the sixth to the tenth weeks, I gave her an herbal pill. But my main concern was her fatigue. Now that she was pregnant, her heart had to work that much harder. I needed to help her get her body stronger.

Around the eighteenth week, Julianna started to exhibit stronger heart palpitations. We modified her acupuncture treatment to include point HT7 and also ear-Shenmen, a point in her ear that is frequently used to calm anxiety and palpitations. This change proved helpful; her heart palpitations became much milder and less frequent. She delivered a beautiful baby girl three days past her due date.

I was—and am—grateful that both daughter and mother were healthy. I am also grateful that Julianna came to see me when she did. Had she been much older before trying to have children, I think it would have been more difficult for her not only to get pregnant but also to hold the pregnancy because of her heart issues. Even if she had managed to bring a child into the world, her energy would have been greatly diminished. I have continued to take care of her after her pregnancy. She will require a regular strengthening regimen of natural therapies.

There are so many hidden things in your body, things you don't know. I was very humbled a few months ago when I went back to see Dr. Dao. I thought I would just go through this again. . . . And all of a sudden, I fell back into that way of thinking that I was perfect. I was planning my cycle, my pregnancy. . . . After all, hadn't I done it once before? I got pregnant—then miscarried.

I was disappointed and went through this whole humbling experience. I was so ungrateful, taking it for granted. Dao basically brought me back to the center. We are trying again now.

I am going into nursing now. I believe in complementary medicine. Western doctors do what they do very well. Unfortunately, they also don't treat the patient as a whole person. They treat your problem on a grand scale, based on a generality of what happens to people. The most frustrating thing about Western medicine is trying to remind them you're you, a whole person. You should have seen what it was like when I was five. The surgery was done by one of the pioneers in the field. My mother later told me: "If your dad and I hadn't been standing just outside the door, we wouldn't have been able to speak to him after the surgery. He had an entourage, and he had no time for you. You were this little morsel for him."

But what I've learned, from my experience with Dao is that every body is different. Every body will react in a different way. I want to learn Western medicine so I can incorporate it with other forms of treatment. I want to work with people and be able to tell them: "Do this treatment before that procedure."

This is where I am. It's the journey.

UNEXPLAINED

Each time, I was always so hopeful. It had to work; it was going to work. The day you get your period, you're devastated. I realized there was something more . . . something we weren't doing. But during that time, while I was taking the Clomid and doing the inseminations, I believed. I was hopeful. And there was reason to be. Every time the doctor would look at the egg, it was perfect. One egg, a couple . . . it all looked so ideal. So why wasn't it working?—Lily

Let's say a woman comes to me as a patient and everything about her health is perfect. She ovulates on time; she has great lubrication; her hormones are stable and at good levels. She's been prodded, inspected, and checked from the inside out by her doctor. She's taken all the tests known to conventional medicine and passed them with flying colors. There are no tubal blockages, no complicating factors; all is as it should be. There's only one problem—she can't get pregnant.

The conventional medical definition of unexplained infertility is simply this: we cannot tell you why you can't get pregnant. Scientifically, we can't find a cause. True, certain factors might figure into it—age, for one. We do know that the number one factor of infertility is age, especially after a woman turns thirty-five. But no one can tell you for sure if age is the cause.

Generally women falling into this unexplained category seem to be normal as defined by conventional medicine. But in traditional Chinese medicine, we look at the subtleties until gradually a much different picture emerges.

If you are not getting pregnant, something is not normal. As I've said, age is a big factor. But there are many other possibilities. Maybe you are not ovulating correctly. Maybe the lining in your uterus is weak. We look for little hints. Has there been a change in your menstrual flow? Is there an increase or decrease in the number of clots? Are there any aspects of your general health that can be improved?

In the clinical medical approach, when we deal with things we can't see, we call them unexplained. In reality, there is always a reason. My job as a traditional Chinese medicine practitioner is to put all the hints together and come up with a probability. Medical care is not always absolute. That's why we must learn to manage uncertainty.

Lily's Story

Lily was forty-one years old when she came to see me. She and her second husband had been trying to get pregnant for a few years.

I made my first mistake, like a lot of people do. But with my ex-husband, having children wasn't an issue. Anyway, I ended up divorcing him.

When George asked me to marry him, I said yes. By then I was in my mid-thirties, and I got engaged right away. But I felt I had to ask: Do I need to decide now if I want to have a child of my own? Do I need to make a decision?

He told me no, I didn't have to decide anything right away. He told me he trusted my instincts. If I decided I wanted to go ahead, he was all right with it. We moved in together and ended up being engaged for two years. We didn't try to get pregnant right away.

And then I hit thirty-eight, and all of a sudden, I wanted a baby. And not just that—it became paramount. I was with the right guy, and my clock was ticking. I guess nature has a way of putting these warning signs up. I remember telling George that I had nothing in common with any of the women in our neighborhood because I didn't have a child. My entire focus took a huge turn.

I had more sex, but there were so many things I didn't know. I didn't know when I ovulated or the best time to get pregnant. I was also a long-distance runner. I didn't know it could affect my fertility until my doctor told me to stop.

Instead, I cut back to five miles a day. That, to me, was stopping. So it was no surprise when six months had passed and I still wasn't pregnant.

I started doing the ovulation kits and taking my temperature every morning. I remember doing it all in secret so my husband wouldn't know. He was fine with me getting pregnant. But it was a whole different thing if I suddenly wanted to do it just because it was ovulation day. It was more my choice than his, I guess. I needed to keep what I was doing private.

Lily had used Clomid for four cycles in conjunction with insemination. Each time, quite a number of follicles developed. And yet she couldn't get pregnant.

The truth was, I was flat-out exhausted by now. I was tired from it, tired of trying to figure it out. Right around this time, my friend called. He had a friend who had gone to an acupuncturist and she ended up pregnant within two months. I had been trying for over a year by this time, and she had gotten pregnant in two months—on her own—with just the acupuncture.

I decided to go see Dr. Dao.

The doctor who had been treating Lily considered her infertility unexplained. When I saw Lily, I saw a woman who had a cycle that was gradually decreasing in two specific ways. Whereas her cycle had once lasted for as long as twenty-seven days, it had been gradually decreasing. By the time she came to me, her cycle was only twenty-three days. Her menstrual flow had also changed—there was a decrease in the amount of blood lost. In addition, she was experiencing night sweats in the days leading up to her period. These premenstrual night sweats can be a telltale sign of decreasing female hormone levels, especially when it comes to estrogen. In fact, tests did indicate a less than ideal FSH level. All of these signs pointed to diminishing fertility.

Lily didn't want to do IVF—she made that clear. She knew it was very hard on the body. She wanted to seek a natural way of getting pregnant.

By then I had had all the tests, and everything looked good. I had stopped running and felt my body change from my running body to my woman body. According to Western medicine, everything was good to go. When I first went to Dr. Dao's office, he didn't suggest more tests. What I remember is him looking at my hand and my tongue, and taking my pulse.

When I looked at Lily's tongue, I saw that there was caking on the surface. This usually indicates a deficiency of blood, fluid, or essence. Her pulse was also very thin. A thin pulse is like a thread. What I wanted was a pulse with a little more volume, more three-dimensional in character. Instead, what I found told me that her blood volume was low, and that she might be prone to anemia and poor blood circulation.

Lily told me she was a long-distance runner. She also mentioned that she had chronic lower back pain, which had troubled her for eight years. Such pain is an issue when it comes to fertility. In Chinese medicine, lower back pain means that endocrine function is weak. It also denotes weak blood flow. So she was symptomatic in several ways: she had a lighter menstrual flow, earlier menstruation, pronounced PMS including food cravings and bloating, and she had this chronic back pain.

And yet she insisted she felt fine.

I am always positive. I knew Chinese medicine and acupuncture had worked for the other woman. I had no reason to believe it wouldn't work for me.

"I feel young," Lily told me. "Why shouldn't I be able to get pregnant? It's not like I feel like I am twenty-one years old, but I certainly don't feel forty-one. I am normal. I haven't aged a lot."

As I looked at her, this is not what I saw. I explained to her that her body was telling her things, but she hadn't yet learned to listen. It was telling her that it needed to get better before she could get pregnant. I told her I saw things that were not normal—like her back pain, for one. Why should she have back pain at forty-one, especially when she was a strong long-distance runner who was so proud of her "conditioning"? Even if she were older, back pain was not necessarily normal.

I knew there were certain things we had to do. I had to strengthen her, first and foremost, despite her insistence that her energy was fine. It was weak, just as her pulse was. I customized a Chinese herbal formula to bolster her blood and her essence. My goal was to improve her egg quality. She was a runner; that meant she scattered her energy around. I included herbs to bring her energy back in.

The formula included angelica root, jujuba fruit, polygoni root, licorice, astragali root, lycii fruit, wheatgrass, and hawthorne berries. I also included dried Chinese mulberry fruit, which is an astringent like blueberries. It's a little sour, not sweet. I chose astringent-quality herbs to try to keep her energy in, to help her rebuild her vitality.

We started treatment in July. Lily followed the program carefully. She would cook these dry herbs into a form of tea and drink it three times a day. She would also come into my clinic for weekly acupuncture treatments. I inserted needles into the areas where she had back pain, as well as points located in her upper back, legs, and the top of her head. The idea was to treat her lower back pain as well as her decreasing fertility. I chose these specific points to increase her blood flow and to stimulate the nerves leading to her lower reproductive system (i.e., the ovaries, fallopian tubes, uterus, cervix, and vagina). One particular point on the top of her head had a dual effect: it not only treated her back pain by inducing endorphin releases into her body, it also regulated her endocrine functions related to the pituitary and the hypothalamus glands.

I started doing treatments. For me, that meant no sugar, no cold liquids. I did everything he said. I was pretty fanatical. I figured I would do exactly what he wanted. I followed everything to the letter. The truth is, I loved going to Dr. Dao. I loved being more healthy. I loved drinking the tea, even though I hated the taste. It was achieving my goal. I was finally heading in the right direction.

After twenty-five days, Lily got her period. It was the first period she'd had since we started working together. By August, her period came after twenty-six days.

I remember feeling wonderful. What made the difference? There was that sense that my body changed because I stopped running.

It was only after treating Lily for weeks that I found out she was not only a runner but a surfer. A surfer! Now the lower back pain made sense. I told her the pain was from being in the cold water. I knew it wasn't going to get better on its own. I had to try a stronger acupuncture treatment for her lower back. By the beginning of October, the back pain started to improve. She also had fewer postovulatory sweats than previously.

My period was late. Something just felt different. I remember flying to see a friend on the East Coast on what would have been day thirty of my cycle. I took a pregnancy test—turns out it was positive. I had to wait another two or three days to confirm with a blood test that I actually was pregnant. It was really something else!

Lily was pregnant and understandably elated. But she still had night sweats, which concerned me. So I added an herb to strengthen her pregnancy. She also had her thyroid levels tested, and they were a little low. She started feeling a little queasy. There was also some pelvic activity, though nothing out of the ordinary. But she was exhausted, more than I would have liked.

You know, when you are pregnant, you feel your age. Because she'd been a runner and a surfer, Lily's body had little energy to hold onto. Her athletic strength was not the kind of strength she needed to support herself and her baby in pregnancy. She had low body fat because her blood and body were crying out to be nourished. In time, they were. Her thyroid got better. That's how she got pregnant.

I was a high-risk pregnancy—and forty-two. I kept following Dr. Dao's diet. I stopped the caffeine—in fact, to this day, I don't drink it. The first month I was okay. But then, in the second month, I started feeling really sick.

Lily's progesterone was a little low. I recommended that she start progesterone supplementation, and her physician agreed. He prescribed the progesterone, which she took throughout her first trimester. As a result, her progesterone levels stabilized. The only problem was that she was extremely nauseous. By the eleventh week of her pregnancy, I switched her from herbal tea to herbal pills.

I went to Dr. Dao, who told me to go out and buy a hamburger. A hamburger! He explained that since I was a vegetarian, what protein I was getting was going to my baby. I felt exhausted and nauseous, so I followed his advice. I went straight to Carl's Jr. on the way home and ordered a hamburger. As soon as I ate it, I immediately felt better. I ate a hamburger every day for a month after that. I even started eating poultry and seafood.

Lily continued to feel tired. I took her pulse in mid-January and suspected she was carrying a girl. Her amniocentesis confirmed it. She still had night sweats, which worried me—no wonder she was tired. I kept my eye on her every week, worrying about a possible miscarriage because of her weak endocrine status. But by nineteen weeks, she was better. She conquered her weakness during the first half of her pregnancy. She ate that burger. She got her energy back.

We wanted to be pregnant so badly. If I had a bad day, all I had to remember was how lucky we were. Eve was born on my mother's birthday. She was born naturally, without any drugs. I wanted to have an epidural, but by the time the doctor arrived, she was out. Eve came a month and three days early. She weighed five pounds, twelve ounces. She was just ready to come.

To me, there's no question in my mind that I became pregnant because of going to see Dr. Dao. Within four months, I was pregnant. And my age was certainly an issue. I believe in him. In fact, I sent two friends to see him.

I would tell anyone to try it, even if you don't know much about it. I had heard about this kind of medicine, but I know that a lot of people haven't. It is almost like hocus pocus to them. You tell someone about this and they're like . . . really? I got pregnant without IVF. I still find that so amazing.

I realize my story had a happy ending. But the process was tough. There are differences in having children at different stages of your life—huge differences. You get to enjoy yourself and your child more. You're older; you have more financial security. Most of all, you have more patience to bring to a child.

MALE

In the past, women have tended to be the primary focus when dealing with matters of infertility. But now, thanks to advances in medicine and science, we have a better understanding of the role that the male plays in many of the challenges facing infertile couples. In fact, abnormalities in men probably appear in somewhere between 30 to 40 percent of infertile couples, making male infertility an important part of reproductive issues.

When dealing with the male challenge, there's one main thing that needs to be considered: sperm. However, there are several aspects of

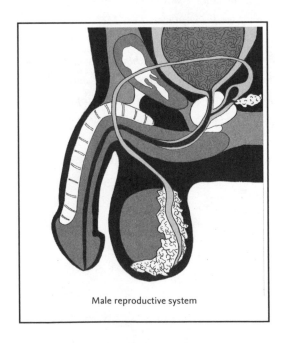

Male reproductive system

> ## Women's Voices
>
> "Who cares whose issue it is? It's both your issue if you're not getting pregnant. You have to be willing to do what it takes. A lot of people don't have that kind of relationship."

sperm quality that figure into the equation, all of which can be uncovered by a simple analysis. *Sperm count* refers to the number of sperm found in semen. A normal sample from a single ejaculation contains at least 40 million sperm. A lower count doesn't mean the man is necessarily infertile; however, it may take longer for conception. *Motility* refers to the ability of the sperm to swim fast enough and straight enough through the cervical mucus to the fallopian tubes to achieve fertilization. Normal sperm motility is about 50 percent. *Morphology* refers to the size and shape of the sperm. Morphology is critical to fertilization, because abnormally shaped sperm might have difficulty swimming or penetrating the egg. For the sperm to be viable, at least 15 percent or more of the sample should be normal. *Concentration* measures the number of sperm cells found in semen. A normal concentration is 20 million sperm per milliliter. Finally, *speed* refers to the number of sperm that are swimming the fastest, giving them the greatest likelihood of reaching the egg for fertilization.

Sperm quality, much like egg quality, can be affected by many different things. For example, alcohol, smoking, and drugs—especially marijuana—all can have a strong effect on sperm quality. Age can also play a part, as sperm concentration and quality start to decline as a man gets older. Stress is another factor; toxins in the environment are another. Men who work in radiation environments such as X-ray labs, or who deal with heavy metals, solvents, and pesticides on a regular basis, are at risk when it comes to maintaining a strong, healthy sperm count.

In Chinese medicine, we believe that sperm issues are a serious factor for men because sperm quality tells us a lot about a man's overall health.

For example, if the sperm concentration is weak, that tells us that the vitality of the man might be poor, or that circulation is an issue. Barring more serious problems (which must be uncovered by further urological testing), the first approach is to begin with a man's lifestyle. We evaluate stress, environment, and overall health—including any chronic illnesses or infections—and then devise a course of herbs and acupuncture. Usually we ask a man to undergo three months of weekly treatments because the sperm production cycle is quite long—approximately seventy-two days. In more than 50 percent of the cases, we see positive changes in the semen parameters following treatment—sometimes as much as 75 percent.

That said, the ratio of men to women seeking treatment for infertility is very small. One reason is that most male factors can be alleviated simply by using insemination. Another option, if the couple is already using IVF, is ICSI (intracytoplasmic sperm injection), in which a single sperm is injected into an egg. Donor sperm is another possibility. Yet the greatest single reason why men don't seek treatment may be attributed to their psychology.

In general, men are not very open to treatments. They'd rather take supplements or vitamins than actually have to face going to a doctor. It's the nature of who men are. Compared to women, they are more afraid of pain; they also don't like to take care of themselves unless something

---

Women's Voices

"I was amazed at how willing my husband was to undergo a vasectomy reversal. That was Western medicine, I guess. There was a surgeon and an operation. But the minute I suggested he come with me for acupuncture treatments, he refused. He didn't mind if I went—probably would have held my hand if I had asked him to—but he wouldn't even consider having acupuncture treatments himself, even if it meant the IVF treatment had a better chance of succeeding."

is going very wrong. Most of the time with semen issues, there are no symptoms. There's no reason for men to suspect that something might be wrong. And the truth is that they don't want to know something is wrong. When it comes to infertility, men don't want to be the problem. In a way, technology has made this possible, because with so many options for women, men don't need to be treated. What's left then is the emotional issue.

In Chinese medicine, we believe that the man is as important as the woman in the partnership required to make a baby. It's important that the man provide love, understanding, and support to his partner. Infertility is one of the biggest challenges for any relationship. It can break up a relationship, or it can make it stronger.

Most of the time in my practice, I see the woman alone. If I could tell men one thing now, it would be this: Don't be passive. Participate. Go to the doctor with your partner, listen to her, and try to understand what she is feeling. Don't feel you have to solve the problem. We know now that intimacy helps increase fertility. So, in the end, it comes to this: just love her.

Part Four

A
NEW BEGINNING

As Life's Gate opens and closes
In the performance of birth and death,
Can you maintain the receptive, feminine principle?
When yin and yang are changing?
After achieving the crystal clear mind,
Can you remain detached and innocent?
Give birth to and nourish all things
Without desiring to possess them.
Give of yourself,
Without expecting something in return.
Assist people, but do not attempt to control them.
This is how to realize the deep virtue of the universe.

—FROM *THE COMPLETE WORKS OF LAO TZU*
TRANSLATION AND ELUCIDATION BY HUA-CHING NI

PREGNANT AT LAST

All of creation has a common beginning.
This common beginning
Is the Mysterious Mother of all.

FROM *THE COMPLETE WORKS OF LAO TZU,*
TRANSLATION AND ELUCIDATION BY HUA-CHING NI

The Monkey King and his little band of fellow travelers finally reached India. The journey had taken so long that it felt like one thousand years had passed. The Monkey King was tired but pleased to have achieved his goal. He had grown in many ways. He had matured and learned humility and patience. All the members of his group had received some form of transformation in their nature and in their being. They had become enlightened spirits. They had always had the power within them, but now they knew how to use it. With the sacred scripture in their hands and with their newfound power, the Monkey King and his entourage flew back to the Chinese Court. What had taken years was now accomplished in the span of a heartbeat.

Now you are pregnant and the long journey seems like a dream. But the journey is far from over. You still have nine to ten more months to keep yourself healthy so that your baby is safe and nourished while waiting to meet you in the outside world. Nine to ten months of anticipation and pure happiness—at least that's what others tell you, especially those who know how long and hard you have traveled to come to this point. That's what you tell yourself. And yet . . .

The truth is that pregnancy is both an exciting and anxiety-producing

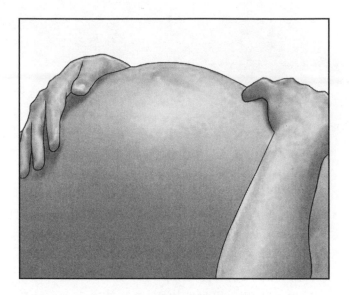

experience, especially if you have suffered miscarriage. A part of you cannot forget that not all pregnancies end in a baby. And yet there is joy and hope. With pregnancy come many dramatic physical and emotional changes. Some women sail through pregnancy with no significant difficulty. Others face challenges. How do you know what your own pregnancy holds for you? Like everything else in life, there are no guarantees. But there are certain factors that can help determine whether you may be facing an easy or a difficult pregnancy.

It all begins with genetics. By looking back at your mother's pregnancy history and experience, it's possible to get some idea of the path your pregnancy may take. Evaluating your lifestyle and health provides you with another window. If you've made it this far, you may have learned that certain habits—such as drinking alcohol, smoking, consuming too much sugar and caffeine, experiencing too much stress—have a strong negative effect on your fertility. The same lessons apply to your pregnancy.

There's another thing we know to be true: a difficult first pregnancy, especially when marked by nausea and vomiting, is a likely indicator of a difficult subsequent pregnancy. So much for the randomness of the universe. Fortunately, Chinese medicine has been used for centuries to relieve many symptoms and prevent complications during pregnancy:

nausea, gestational diabetes, preeclampsia, fibroids, lower back pain, low fetal weight, and miscarriage—just to name a few. Whether through a program of herbal treatments or acupuncture or the two in combination, Chinese medicine can be an effective and safe tool for the successful management of pregnancy symptoms. The best part? No ill side effects to you or to the baby you are carrying.

Women's Voices

"Dr. Dao did light massage around my neck and back when he took the needles out. The baby responded to the acupuncture treatments, too. When I lay there, the baby would get extremely active, kicking and punching, while the needles were in. It was a great feeling."

Eating for a healthy pregnancy involves the same principles of healthy nutrition during other times of your life. There are three fundamental principles: safety, variety, and feasibility. Eating foods that are fresh, without traces of pesticides, chemical fertilizers, and heavy metals, should be the most important step during this time. This means eating more organic foods and fewer packaged and preserved foods. It also means heeding local fishery advisories and not overconsuming fish that might be high in trace heavy metals. Finally, it means eating much less raw food unless you are certain that a given food is free of contaminants. Of course, for all sushi lovers, this means taking a hiatus from raw fish.

Eating a greater variety of foods can ensure a better nutrient spectrum for your baby. Better eating means better fetal growth and development. One of the best things you can eat during this time is dark green leafy vegetables. Don't limit yourself to one kind—you'll be surprised to learn just how many different varieties of these nutrient-rich vegetables there are.

Besides developing pregnancy sickness with nausea and even vomiting, many pregnant women find they develop unique taste sensitivities that limit their appetite for certain foods. That's why it's important to prepare foods in ways that make them easy to digest. For some women, this could mean eating more soup and semiliquid foods. For others, it could mean eating dryer and more solid foods like toast. Eating smaller portions more frequently has been found to be very helpful for the majority of my pregnant patients.

Below are some suggestions for healthy eating throughout these all-important months of pregnancy. Not everyone has the same tastes, of course, but everyone needs good nutrition—especially your developing baby. The portions below are just a guide. You will need to eat more or less depending on your baby's needs as you progress in your pregnancy.

A Healthy Eating Plan for Pregnancy

Breakfast Choices

Rice porridge
Combine ½ cup of cooked brown rice with 1½ cups of water and bring to a boil. Turn down the heat and simmer, adding slices of ginger and salt to taste. Cook until the rice porridge is slightly thick. This dish is very bland and great for morning sickness. You may have the porridge with a side dish of vegetables, or top with pine nuts, walnuts, dried figs, or apple slices.

Barley cereal
In a saucepan or crock pot, combine ¼ cup of barley, ¼ cup of barley flakes, ¼ cup of millet, 10 Chinese jujube dates, and 1 slice of fresh ginger with 3½ cups of water. Cook in a crock pot overnight or on the stovetop for 2½ to 3 hours on low, stirring occasionally.

Scrambled tofu
4–5 ounces of tofu scrambled with diced zucchini and mushrooms or finely chopped celery and tomato. Season with 1 tablespoon of tamari soy sauce; beverage: 1 cup of lemon tea

1 poached egg, 1 slice of whole-grain toast, with 2 slices of turkey bacon
   or chicken sausage; beverage: 1 cup of chamomile tea
1 cup of any cooked whole-grain cereal served hot with 1 teaspoon of
   vanilla extract stirred in, topped with slices of banana or strawberries;
   beverage: 1 cup of organic unsweetened soy milk
1 large organic hard-boiled egg with slices of avocado and 1 slice of
   whole-grain toast with 2 tablespoons of hummus spread on top; beverage: 6 ounce serving of fresh organic orange juice

Protein cereal
Soak 1 cup of brown rice, ⅓ cup of soybeans, and 1 tablespoon of black
sesame or sunflower seeds in hot water for 2 hours. Pour into a blender
and blend well. Pour into a saucepan and cook on the stovetop over low
heat for 1 to 2 hours. Add more hot water if needed during this cooking
process.

Lunch/Dinner Choices
Lentil soup made with chicken or vegetable broth (canned or boxed
   broth is fine, as long as it is organic) and chopped carrots, celery, and
   mushrooms
1 medium cubed sweet potato or yam and chopped kale sautéed in
   chicken or vegetable broth with toasted sesame oil lightly drizzled
   on top
4–5 ounces of baked or grilled wild salmon seasoned with salt and pepper
   and lemon with a side of mashed yams and steamed asparagus
4–5 ounces of steamed sole or catfish with ½ cup fermented black beans
   (can be purchased in oriental markets or at Whole Foods) and 1 tablespoon of tamari soy sauce with a side of basmati rice and cooked
   spinach
Chicken noodle soup made with cooked organic chicken, shiitake mushrooms, carrots, napa cabbage, green onions, egg noodles and 2 slices
   of ginger
Beef noodle soup made with thinly sliced organic beef, beef broth, bok
   choy, green onions, and rice noodles or egg noodles, garnished with
   cilantro

Nourishing herbal chicken soup
Combine these ingredients in a crock pot: 1 organic chicken breast, 2 organic chicken thighs (all with bone), 9 grams of angelica (dang gui), 6 grams of rehmannia (shou di), 10 grams of pseudostellaris (haung qi), 3 grams of licorice root (gan cao), 4 pieces of Chinese jujube dates (da zao), and 4½ cups of water. Cook for 3 hours. Discard the herbs when the soup is done. (*Note:* You can also use a Dutch oven or a heavy metal pot. Bring all ingredients to a boil, then simmer on low heat for 4 or more hours, until chicken is tender.)

Follow your same supplement regimen as when you were trying to get pregnant. A good formula of prenatal vitamins containing adequate amounts of folic acid, calcium, iron, and DHA will also be helpful.

A Healthy Exercise Program for Pregnancy

Exercise should be gentle during pregnancy. Stick with exercises that you are used to and try not to start any new programs of exercise during pregnancy. The only exception is swimming. If your pregnancy has created a lot of discomfort in your body, you might find swimming or doing aquatic exercises helpful. To that end, I usually recommend that patients increase their exercise regimen as they near the end of their pregnancy. Undertaking more exercise near the end of the pregnancy can usually decrease complications and help the delivery process to go more smoothly.

The Chinese believe that when your baby is born, it is already nearly one year old by the lunar calendar. That means that your life with this baby exists from the moment you get pregnant. This next part of your journey is all about fetal education. Besides taking care of your body by eating good food and exercising, you should also enrich your spirit. Your baby is very much connected to your sensory organs. Whenever there is an overwhelming sensory input, your baby can feel it. Therefore, listen to good music, and stay away from anything too jarring or loud or melancholy. The same principle applies to books. Read things that are happy and uplifting, with good stories infused with creativity and life. Stay away from things that make you feel anxious or frightened or sad.

Trying so hard to get pregnant can create anxiety. For some, that anxiety doesn't go away easily, especially if you have a history of miscarriage. In those moments when you need to find peace of heart, reflect on your blessing. Let it calm you and help you to anticipate with joy the child who awaits you.

MOTHERHOOD
AND BEYOND

Give birth and nourish all things
Without desiring to possess them.
Give of yourself,
Without expecting something in return.

FROM *THE COMPLETE WORKS OF LAO TZU,*
TRANSLATION AND ELUCIDATION BY HUA-CHING NI

Motherhood is frequently a new beginning for many women. It fulfills a sense of purpose, and it is the highest form of duty and honor for the propagation of the human race. Regardless of how many children you have, a child teaches you to be kind, compassionate, and loving. Children teach all of us that the most important things are not fame and fortune but intimacy and family. You will accumulate knowledge and wisdom that you can share with other women. Everything you will learn in motherhood applies to our world. How can we bring this beautiful energy of mothering to our world so that we can have fewer wars and more harmony in learning to live with each other? I firmly believe that this world can be a better place if we all respect and learn from the energetic wisdom of mothering. Once you are a mother, you will be a mother forever. You will teach your children and others to care just a little more about each other and to embrace differences among people. You will bring this energy forth to share with others so that you are truly a mother of the world.

Postpartum Health

There are nearly four million childbirths in the United States each year. Yet postpartum care is often neglected by the medical profession as well as by our culture. You dutifully take your baby for a two-week checkup and then monthly checkups; but at the most, you see your doctor once after delivery, usually at your six-week checkup. All that time and effort put into monitoring you and your baby while you are pregnant—but once your baby leaves your womb, it is a different story. You are the single most important part of your baby's world, the very center of your baby's universe. And yet, with the attention shifting to the infant, the health state of the mother takes a back seat.

Giving—isn't that what motherhood is all about? But how can you give when you are depleted and not taking proper care of yourself? What most people don't realize is that the consequence of neglecting your own health needs will result in weakness. That weakness will, from the Chinese medical perspective, sow the seeds for future illnesses such as degenerative diseases that may come soon or may not manifest for another decade or two. This is especially the case when women use stimulating drugs and advanced reproductive technology in their quest to become pregnant. Remember my caution in earlier chapters about the consequences of fighting nature? Older women may have beaten the odds by having children late in life, but that doesn't mean nature won't retaliate in some form if you don't take proper care of yourself after your baby is born.

I can imagine you protesting, "But I did the hard part: I had a healthy baby! And now you're telling me I'm not out of the woods?" That's exactly what I am saying. Certain things happen in the immediate aftermath of childbirth. Among the symptoms you most likely will experience are fatigue, poor sleep, depression, and anxiety. There can be breast-feeding complications; there can be problems with uterine bleeding and even arthritis.

Chinese medicine practitioners believe that pregnancy and childbirth can deplete vital qi (energy) and blood. They weaken the kidney and spleen systems and exhaust the jing (essence), which makes the body vulnerable to attacks of pathogenic factors; that is, disease conditions that have been lying in wait in your body will finally find a pathway through your exhausted system. If you are young and healthy, you most likely will do just fine. If you are older but healthy, you may still do just fine. But if you are unhealthy with chronic illnesses, regardless of how old you are, you might develop new health problems or your chronic problems may get worse. It is therefore essential to be on the outlook for any symptoms and signs and address them immediately.

The first month after the delivery is a critical time for both mother and child. While the infant has just entered a new world and the baby's systems are quite fragile, the mother is also entering a new role, perhaps including breast-feeding, and is still bleeding from the labor process. As a new mother, you are particularly vulnerable as you learn to cope with the burden of taking care of a baby. In Chinese and many other cultural traditions, new mothers and newborns are advised to stay comfortable at home as much as possible for the first month, avoiding outings other than seeing doctors. Only the closest relatives or friends who take care of the baby are allowed to see the baby for the first month. These precautions are meant to avoid the transmission of any possible infectious illnesses.

After labor, immediate strenuous exercises are to be avoided since your "inside" is still raw and weak from the labor process. Taking a bath should also be refrained from until your bleeding has completely stopped, usually four to six weeks after delivery. Try to rest around the baby's schedule. Good rest and nutrition at this time will not only ensure your breast milk to be of the highest quality if you breast-feed, but it can also help you recover better and faster without complications such as postpartum depression.

Many of our patients ask for specific postpartum dietary guidance. In general, the same eating principles apply here as during other times of life: eat healthy, eat well, and do not skip meals. My colleagues and I at Tao of Wellness have come up with a general meal menu as a reference. Obviously this only serves as a guide and you can modify it as you see fit for your circumstances. The meals are not only nutritious but are meant to nourish your body after the exertion of labor and the subsequent loss of blood from childbirth. This menu is also a good way to prepare you for the task of breast-feeding, should you so choose.

Postpartum Menu (If You Are Breast-feeding)

Days 1–7

You can eat a regular diet without restriction. However, you should avoid cold drinks and raw foods.

After Day 7

Breakfast Choices

2 organic eggs scrambled with green onions and 2–3 ounces of sliced turkey; beverage: a 6-ounce serving of fresh orange juice

Cabbage porridge
Combine these ingredients in a saucepan: ½ cup of shredded cabbage, ½ cup of cooked brown rice, 2 cups of water, pinch of salt, ¼ cup of cilantro, 3 ounces of shredded chicken. Bring to a boil over high heat, then reduce heat to medium-low and cook until slightly thick.

1 cup of warm oat bran cereal mixed with 1 cup of warm organic un-sweetened soy milk, topped with a handful of mixed berries and slices of half a banana

1 to 2 slices of whole-grain toast with organic almond butter served with ½ cup of fresh strawberries; beverage: a 6-ounce serving of fresh orange juice

Choose a breakfast option from the non–breast-feeding menu on pages 224 and 225.

Lunch/Dinner Choices

1 cup of cooked millet or quinoa served with sautéed mustard greens and 3–4 ounces of firm tofu, with toasted sesame oil, shredded nori (seaweed), and black sesame seeds sprinkled on top

4–5 ounces of sliced lean beef or chicken sautéed with basil and mint on 1 cup of brown rice; medley of steamed cauliflower, carrots, and snow peas

4–5 ounces of baked or steamed red snapper; spinach or kong xin cai (a type of Chinese vegetable called "empty heart") sautéed or steamed with ginger and a pinch of salt

4–5 ounces of grilled or baked chicken breast seasoned with cumin, black pepper, and paprika; ½ cup black beans, sautéed spinach, and shallots

Dandelion soup with brown rice

Make the broth out of dandelion greens, using just the leafy plant part. Chop and add to a pot of water with a little chopped onion, celery, and carrot tops and a pinch of salt. Then add 1 cup of cooked brown rice (or cooked barley) into the broth (you may choose to eat the dandelion or remove it along with the carrot tops and other vegetables).

Black Sesame Oil Chicken Soup (see Appendix: Recipes, page 242) with rice noodles or brown rice

Drunken Shrimp (see Appendix: Recipes, pages 242 and 243) with snow peas and ½ cup of whole-grain pasta

Mixed bean soup

Combine 3 or 4 different types of beans, soak overnight or for 2 hours in hot water, discard the soaking water. Add new water, chopped carrots, tomato, potato, fennel seeds, bay leaf, and celery. Bring to a boil, then turn down the heat and simmer until the beans are tender, about 1 hour.

Non–Breast-Feeding Diet

Breakfast Choices

2 organic eggs fried in 1½ tablespoons of sesame oil, served with 1 slice of whole-grain toast with 4 slices of avocado; beverage: 1 cup of warm soy organic milk

2 organic eggs (any style) served with 1 slice of whole-grain toast with hummus and a few slices of tomato; beverage: 1 cup of warm organic soy milk

2 organic eggs scrambled with ½ teaspoon of sesame oil, ½ teaspoon of olive oil, chopped spinach, and mushrooms; beverage: 1 cup of green tea.

Tonic Cereal (see Appendix: Recipes, page 243)

Black Bean/Brown Rice Cereal (see Appendix: Recipes, page 243)

Mao's Cereal (available at www.taoofwellness.com)

1 cup of any whole-grain warm cereal topped with mixed berries, 4–5 dried figs or 2–3 fresh figs, and 1 cup of warm soy milk (you may drink the soy milk by itself or mixed with the cereal)

2 large whole-grain blueberry pancakes lightly drizzled with fresh organic maple syrup; beverage: 1 cup of almond milk

Lunch/Dinner Choices

Black Sesame Oil Chicken Soup (see Appendix: Recipes, page 241) with rice noodles or brown rice

Herbal Chicken or Lamb Soup (see Appendix: Recipes, page 244)

3–4 ounces of tofu and basil sautéed with 2 tablespoons of sesame oil, steamed Chinese broccoli (drizzle with 1 tablespoon of soybean paste when ready to serve), and 1 cup of cooked brown rice

4–5 ounces of tilapia steamed with 2 tablespoons of tamari soy sauce, 1 tablespoon of sesame oil, and several slices of ginger; steamed or sautéed broccoli and brown rice

1 medium yam with sautéed mustard greens and ½ pound of diced tofu

Drunken Shrimp (see Appendix: Recipes, pages 242 and 243) with whole-grain pasta

Ginger clam soup

In a large pot, combine 1 pound of clams, 1 cup of water, 4 slices of fresh ginger, and a pinch of salt. Cover pot and bring to a boil until the clams open.

1 cup rice and black beans with 4 to 5 ounces of lean sirloin steak and sautéed kale or spinach

Looking from the Other Side: Lessons to Teach Your Child

When you were in your mother's tummy as a fetus, your ovaries contained many eggs. Once you were born, those eggs still numbered in the six digits.

But as time went on, you started to ovulate. The best eggs popped out of the ovaries first. By the time you reached your thirties, lesser-quality eggs were left behind. The equation is fairly simple: The older you are, the more you have ovulated. The more you have ovulated, the poorer the egg quality of those remaining eggs. And if you have any health issues or if your general well-being is less than it should be, it will further affect the viability of these eggs in your ovaries.

The long-held common wisdom was that brain cells—what we call neurons—cannot regenerate once they are lost. Based on recent scientific evidence, we know this is not true. If you have a solid foundation of good nutrition and cell health, you can actually help the brain cells rejuvenate. To a certain extent, the same is true of your eggs. Even though age remains a strong determining factor for your pregnancy outcome, having a healthy body, strong constitution, and relaxed mental perspective can all increase your odds of pregnancy. By the same token, if you are in your twenties but abuse your body with a poor lifestyle, insufficient sleep, excessive amount of stress, smoking and drinking, and dieting to look as thin as a chopstick, this will for certain damage your ovarian reserve, weaken your fertility potential, and even bring on your menopause earlier.

It's ironic—sex education is universally taught in our public systems, often from an early age. But the Western emphasis is traditionally placed on teaching young women how *not* to get pregnant. The problem with this one-sided approach is that many women grow up thinking they know all there is to know about pregnancy and conception, when in reality, all they've learned is pregnancy prevention. We fear that teens will run out and get pregnant early if they know too much about their fertility. But I would argue that knowledge is power. The more we teach teens about their reproductive life—from the time of their first period through the process of menopause—the more they will realize that what they do at an early age can affect their chances of getting pregnant later. Let them understand their fertility; let them treasure and nurture it.

The bottom line is that the more you can do to keep yourself healthy, the better your fertility potential. This is the lesson you should be teaching your children, starting from an early age.

22

WHEN DREAMS DON'T
COME TRUE

Dealing with Loss

Loss is natural. There is birth and death in life. Loss occurs every day, in every living organism. This is a normal process. People go through it; other organisms go through it. It is the cycle of imperfection in the world.

If you believe in God, the seeming randomness of loss can lead you to believe that God is very unfair. But if you look more carefully, this unfairness is actually the fairness of God. Life is meant to have random situations, not all of them easy. Some we can control and some we cannot. Sudden losses, pain, death—whether of a person or of a dream—are situations that help us to grow and to survive. Or not to survive—that is the other choice. This is the way nature is. It rules by checks and balances.

By no means am I downplaying the pain of loss. It hurts. Loss can be great, especially when dealing with infertility. If you lose a child through miscarriage or are not able to become pregnant, it will be imprinted on

Women's Voices

"I went to Dao because I had just gone through a miscarriage. My spirit was so crushed. He helped me realize it was natural. He gave me a realistic picture in an ancient yet modern way. He treated me as a person and not just a uterus—that's what Chinese medicine offers. It allowed me to keep going with my life, even when I was in my deepest despair."

your soul forever. Nothing can erase the memory of loss. It is part of your history.

But dealing with loss doesn't mean you have to accept it. Take death: Psychologists tell us that we have to accept it. But I say be angry, be upset, feel cheated—all that matters is whether you can heal from your loss. You don't have to embrace your pain. Be angry as hell if it helps you. Carry your history and your passions and your emotions with you. As much as you might want time to stand still, it is always moving on. That is what you must do, when you are ready. The healing process is about moving forward with the best energy you can gather. You never know what the future can bring. Life is a challenge. And one of the biggest challenges you can face is living with pain, whether physical, emotional, or spiritual.

Alternatives to Pregnancy: Adoption, Surrogacy, Donor Egg, Living Without Children

When you are trying to become pregnant with your own child, you probably will not give up unless nature fights you so hard that you must stop. In my practice, I have seen women so single-minded about becoming pregnant that alternatives such as donor egg do not interest them at the beginning. Even thinking about these options may seem to be too

> ## Women's Voices
>
> "Infertility is a hard thing to go through. At the fertility clinic, it was all so cut and dried. I kept doing all these treatments. I'd go to the office and see all these women with sad faces. . . . Dao was brutally honest. After a year, he told me it was time to stop. He literally got down on his hands and knees and begged me not to do more IVF. He told me that it wasn't going to happen. Then he brought up the alternatives, telling me there were so many ways to be a mother."

negative and to be avoided in the fear that such thoughts may interfere with getting pregnant with your own egg. But if having a healthy child is the ultimate goal, there are many different ways to achieve it. There are options. You can ultimately become a mother if that is what you choose, if you can just open your eyes to different options.

The ancients had a wonderful take on the idea of openness and finding ways to reach a dream. Look at a vase. The usefulness of the vase is in its empty space, which can be filled with so many things. Lao Tzu teaches us not to look at things in just one way. Life is not linear but circular, and it is filled with many options and paths.

Surrogacy/Donor Eggs

I personally find the processes of surrogacy and donor eggs to be purely amazing. They're all about sharing and are true compassion and humility at work. I hold very high esteem for women who are willing to donate themselves to this process of childbearing, be it by giving their eggs or by sharing their uterus.

Some might argue that because money is involved, egg donors and surrogates are in it for business reasons. But Taoists believe that you always gives something for something in return. That's why I don't have any problem with the money issue. I look at it as an energy exchange. It

> ### Women's Voices
>
> "I did donor because I needed to move on. I have friends on pins and needles, always waiting. . . . But I knew I had to get out of wanting and into *having*. The reason why I feel so complete and fine with my ultimate decision is because I fought the good fight. Was there is a little sadness and mourning? Sure. But it has no effect on how much I love my daughter."

helps create a situation where that child you are helping to create truly becomes yours. It's an energy transaction. If a woman really wants to have the process of a pregnancy and can't do it on her own, I would absolutely recommend she consider this path.

Recently, one of my patients came to me for help in choosing a donor. She showed me pictures of two women. She liked one; her husband liked the other. There was no tangible reason for their preferences, other than how the two women looked. To some degree, we are attracted to certain energies. You can check IQs and SAT scores; you can study the color of a woman's eyes or her hair. At some point, though, you and your partner just go with your gut feeling—assuming the prospective donor is young, with no major bad habits or troublesome genetic history.

Put it this way: If you had a chance to relive your life, to make healthier choices, to eat well, and to avoid stress and bad habits, wouldn't you do it? That's how you must think of the donor—as a new chance. Take time to investigate all possibilities. Make sure you work with an agency that weeds out women who, either for physical or psychological reasons, are not desirable donors. Talk to the people in the agency; know what criteria they use for selecting donors.

For the most part, surrogates are women who already have children, who choose for financial and altruistic reasons to share their uterus and body. You should consider a woman with a relatively healthy lifestyle, good nutrition practices, and with no bad habits such as smoking, drinking, or use of recreational drugs. You should also inquire if the woman is regularly exposed to secondhand smoke. If these issues are cause for concern, she may not be a good surrogate. While genetic material generally doesn't transfer into the baby, nurturing and living habits do. Surrogacy is usually considered as an option when your uterus or your body is not in a healthy state, where pregnancy might jeopardize your health and the baby's health.

Adoption

When other options are not suitable options for you, adoption should be considered. Adoption raises concerns that many women have to work through. One is the concern that the child doesn't carry your genetics. In addition, you don't know what the mother might have done to compromise her health. For example, did she drink; did she take drugs throughout her pregnancy? Usually adoption agencies have fairly extensive histories of the biological mothers and the family, but there are still many genetic and lifestyle factors that you don't—and won't—know.

To those who worry, I would say this: There is a randomness that is part of life. While it's nice to know genetic information, it's not always helpful and it is not absolutely predictive. Obviously you should seek to know as much as possible. But the reality is that even if you review a relatively complete set of genetic information, there is no way that you could say this child is going to be in any way worse or better than a child with your own genes, because, in a way, everything is randomized. Nothing in the universe is perfect, and that includes all of our offspring. That imperfection is what makes this universe so diverse. If everyone were the same, we would be no better than robots. Everyone's muscles would be the same; everyone's thinking processes would be the same; everyone's nose, eye color, hair . . . all the same. Just think how boring the world would be.

Nature doesn't work that way. Nature is about mixing it up. Remember, nature is about chaos: the interdependence of chaos and order. My desk at home, for example, is frequently chaotic. It never really reaches perfect order. I clean it up only to find it messy again after a while. This cycling of order and chaos is the way of nature. Each creates purpose for the existence of the other. Adoption is like that. It occurs when a mother-to-be is not capable of rearing the child for financial, maturity, and many other possible life reasons. While life is a chaos for this mother, hopefully, in an orderly fashion, another mother-to-be will accept this gift from a fellow human being.

Similarly, every child in the world is perfect because you as the mother can make it so. That's the case whether that child comes from your genes or from someone else's. Thus an adopted child will not be more imperfect than your own child, genetically speaking. The truth is that you can't always know all the so-called red flags in a child's genetic makeup. Your own biological child might carry genes that you don't even know you have. Ironically, sometimes you might end up having more information about a child you adopt that you would about your biological offspring.

There are people who think that there are no coincidences in life and that adopted children are meant to be with certain parents; that the match is predestined or meant to be. Taoists are of this school of thought. Remember yin and yang? Taoists believe that this duality exists in each of us: We think that because we have free will, we are able to do things in any way we like. But, as always, there is the other side of the coin: predetermined destiny. Because we are beings of energy, we are magnets. Like it or not, we will draw certain things into our life, including certain people. And then there is a third factor: the mystery of life. This is what brings a certain amount of randomness. We will always attempt to control our life—that is human nature. But there will be times when certain things will not go our way. And we must learn to accept and appreciate them for the lessons they bring.

When you are born, the stars line up in certain ways. The earth, the magnetic forces, the place where you were born, the family you are with—all of these things and more create an energy dynamic unique to you. But there is also free will. Destiny, free will, and yes, randomness—Taoists believe all are true. How much and how little of each has to do with the interplay of your energy with the energy of this world.

What all this means is simply that you end up with the child you were meant to have. I've heard it said that when you adopt a child, that child becomes your own. I say this: That child is your own and always was. The only difference is the path you did not predict you would take.

Living Without Children

You really don't have to live without children. There are many children who need guidance and help. I know of two couples who don't have children, but the women are Big Sisters who share their time with children from an underprivileged community. Many women and many couples put their effort into helping children by volunteering in schools, at hospitals, and at other places where children need love, hope, and guidance. By putting their energy into helping children, they become part of the parenting process.

Consider teachers—they are part of parenting. In fact, to me, they are parents of an educational sort. They are sharing knowledge and helping children grow up and reach their full potential.

You never have to live without children. Think about what you can give to the world, to the community. You always get more than you give.

IN BALANCE FOR THE
REST OF YOUR LIFE

I anchor my being to that which existed
Before heaven and earth were formed.
I alone am innocent and unknowing,
Like a newborn babe.
Unoccupied by worldly cares,
I move forward to nowhere.

FROM *THE COMPLETE WORKS OF LAO TZU,*
TRANSLATION AND ELUCIDATION BY HUA-CHING NI

Throughout this book, we've looked at the importance of wellness in trying to get pregnant. But wellness doesn't stop with or without a baby; wellness is a lifelong commitment, much like having a child. Wellness means having peace in your heart and having the ability to find joy and contentment in simple things in your life. It is not merely the absence of pain; rather, it is the ability to embrace and accept imbalances while trying to improve a little every day.

No one is in perfect health. But as a woman, you have a body that is complex in design. You went on a journey to have a child. That journey has reached its natural course. Now you are entering a different phase of your life—one no less important than what has come before. A new chapter is to be written. And the care that you have taken in your pursuit of trying to get pregnant can be applied to these days and years that follow.

Perimenopause and Menopause

My practice is full of women in their forties who are trying to get pregnant. Some are already going through the perimenopausal process. Perimenopause is the time before actual menopause when you begin to experience some of the symptoms and signs of menopause. The average age of menopause throughout the world has been consistent for centuries or more. In the United States, it is around fifty-one, and in China, it is around forty-nine.

Interestingly, not everyone experiences perimenopausal or menopausal symptoms. In fact, some women simply stop menstruating without any menopausal symptoms. Then there are women who have every symptom in the book. The same thing holds true for the perimenopausal transition. The symptoms of perimenopause range from mild night sweats or premenstrual hot flashes to multiple symptoms such as changes in menstrual pattern, hot flashes, night sweats, sleep problems, vaginal and skin dryness, mood changes, decreased mental clarity, hair loss or thinning, and decreased libido.

During perimenopause, your endocrine system and your ovaries are starting to weaken, making lower levels of hormones such as estrogen and progesterone. This is a natural signal of your reproductive aging process. Women normally go through perimenopause in their early forties, but some women start perimenopause earlier, even in their thirties. The onset and duration of perimenopause varies from woman to woman. In your thirties and your forties, you move into the perimenopausal transition. This premenopausal period can last anywhere from a few months to several years. It depends on when your mother entered menopause; how well you have taken care of yourself; whether and how much you drink or smoke; and numerous other factors.

Often women ask me how they know when they are in perimenopause. The signs are there: you have only to read them. Take sleep—it is more shallow; are you more restless? Do you find that you are not able to sleep for as long a period of time? Or perhaps you are finding yourself taking more frequent naps. All of these sleep issues can point to perimenopause, especially when occurring premenstrually.

Hot flashes are another sign. So are night sweats, flushes, or intervals when your skin feels warm. Or maybe you see changes in your appearance. Your skin is dryer; your hair is thinner. All of these are signs of change.

Is there is any way to slow down the perimenopause process; that is, is there any treatment for perimenopause? This question is most often on the minds of women who are trying to get pregnant. If that is the case, the answer is that you can sometimes use a natural approach with Chinese herbs and acupuncture to counteract the aging process taking place in your reproductive system. There have even been a few instances where I was able to temporarily reverse a woman's perimenopause in order to help her get pregnant. It ultimately depends on your ovarian reserve, which can be measured only relatively.

If you are not trying to get pregnant but simply want to address some of the symptoms you might be experiencing, the natural approach is still a good one. If that does not work and your symptoms are affecting your quality of life, you may want to consult with your physician. There are frequently two possible solutions. Some women take oral contraceptives to ease perimenopausal symptoms, even if they don't need them for birth control. These hormone treatments of combined estrogen and progestin can help keep your periods regular as well as ease symptoms. Talk with your doctor to see if this option is for you. If you are over thirty-five, you should not take birth-control pills if you smoke or have a history of blood clots. You will need a prescription to get oral contraceptives. Some women begin hormone replacement therapy (HRT) even before menopause. HRT contains much lower doses of hormones than the pill and thus has less risk for bad side effects. However, current studies such as the Women's Health Initiative have advised that women should take hormones only when needed for symptomatic relief, especially of vasomotor symptoms like hot flashes and night sweats.

Making lifestyle changes can also help ease your symptoms and keep you healthy. Just as during all the stages of your life, you must eat healthfully. It's particularly important that you eat to address some of the changes that are going on in your body. For example, one of the greatest risks you face after menopause is osteoporosis (extreme bone loss). Heart disease is another risk. That's why it's crucial to eat lots of whole-grain foods, vegetables, and fruits, and especially to add calcium-rich foods to your diet. Make sure you take a calcium supplement to obtain your recommended daily intake. Get adequate vitamin D from sunshine or a supplement. Avoid alcohol and caffeine, which can trigger hot flashes in some women and can disrupt sleep.

Get moving. Regular exercise helps keep your weight down, helps you sleep better, makes your bones stronger, and boosts your mood status. Try to get at least thirty minutes of exercise most days of the week, but let your doctor recommend what's best for you. Find healthy ways to cope with stress. Try meditation or yoga—both can help you relax, as well as help you handle your symptoms more easily.

Most of all, understand and accept the seasonal changes in your body. We all have a tendency to fight against change—this is human nature. But the road to contentment and inner peace lies in appreciating each new phase of life and the challenges it brings.

Perimenopause is very much like nature at summer's end. The leaves are starting to fall, the temperature cools, and the air turns dryer. As autumn turns to winter, your body turns from the period of fertility to the nonreproductive stage of life. As it should: because you—all of us—cannot be summer forever. Where there is growth, there must be withering. This is the wisdom of nature.

Nobody likes to age. This is especially true in our culture, where youthful appearance and vitality are valued beyond their true worth. The key is to accept gracious aging. Accept what your body can and cannot do. It's no different than when you were young. You knew that if you pushed your body too far, you would hurt yourself. It's about honoring the capabilities unique to each stage of life. You can't stay up all night; you can't drink too much and still expect to just get up and go. The question is: Why would you want to?

Leaving with a Lesson

You are on your way to becoming an elder. I know that may be a frightening thought, but not if you look at it from a larger perspective. In China, elders have lived many years and have a tremendous amount of life experience and wisdom to share. Elders are the most respected population of the entire country. They hold the highest position in every family and in society.

We are, in the balance of the rest of our life, becoming the elder. It's not about aging but about transmitting our wisdom and experience so that future generations will not suffer and will have a better life. This especially applies to mothers—both those who have children and those who have expressed their motherhood by taking this journey.

My father, who is a very wise man, told me something long ago that has stayed in my memory ever since: "To stay young, we must act young." Not immature, but flexible and supple as a baby or small child. Babies are soft; they are moldable. Above all, they are open to the world. They see the beauty and adventure of life.

And so we leave you with a lesson. The Monkey King traveled far to the West, and with his companions, he finally received the sacred scriptures of the work of the Buddha. As a team, they brought this invaluable work back to China and spread the benevolent work of the Buddha to enrich everyone with compassion and a deeper understanding of the meaning of life.

The journey to motherhood is no different from this story. Your companions on your journey can include your partner, your medical professionals, and your closest friends. Your journey is no less difficult, with plenty of challenges and detours. The journey itself will help you in achieving a deeper understanding of your true nature. Perhaps with disappointment you will accept the path of life without a child. Either way, your journey is sure to be an enlightening experience, and in the end, with or without a child, you will have become a mother in your heart and soul. Your wish to extend your spirit to another soul is the fundamental compassionate nature of a true mother. Thus it is that in the end you will find your motherhood in your heart. If we can all learn from this journey as human beings, this world can be filled with more love, compassion, and tolerance for imperfection and for each other. This is the true meaning of humanity.

We hope this book has brought you more clarity. We thank you for allowing us the opportunity to assist you on this wonderful journey.

APPENDIX
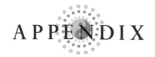

Recipes

Chinese Rice Porridge

½ cup barley
10 grams shan yao (Chinese yam)
5 pieces dao zao (a type of date)
5 cups filtered water

Combine the ingredients in a medium saucepan and quickly bring to a boil. Turn down the flame and simmer until soft (about 1½–2 hours).

Basic Chicken Broth

1 organic chicken (3–4 pounds), cut up with skin on
7 cups filtered water
2 tablespoons salt
2 carrots, chopped
2 stalks of celery, chopped
¼ small head of savoy cabbage, chopped
5 peppercorns
1 teaspoon chopped fresh parsley

Place the chicken in a large stock pot, and add the water and the salt. Bring to a boil over high heat, then reduce heat and simmer for 30 minutes. Add the rest of the ingredients and cook on low heat for an additional 30 minutes. Remove the chicken and strain the broth. Chill the strained broth until the fat separates from the liquid. Skim the fat from the top of the liquid. This broth stays fresh in the refrigerator for 2 days or can be frozen for future use.

Barley Chicken Soup

2 tablespoons olive oil
½ medium sweet onion, chopped
½ shallot, chopped
1 cup chopped celery
2 cloves garlic, minced
1 cup diced red potatoes
3 cups cooked organic chicken, chopped
2½ quarts chicken broth (homemade or organically prepared)
1 cup quick-cooking barley
½ cup chopped fresh parsley
sea salt and black pepper, to taste

Heat the oil in a large stock pot over medium heat. Sauté the sweet onion, shallot, celery, and garlic in the oil under the onions are tender. Mix in the potatoes, chicken, and broth. Bring to a boil, and then stir in the barley. Reduce heat, cover, and simmer for 20 minutes. Remove from heat, stir in the parsley, and season with salt and pepper to taste.

Herbal Organic Chicken Soup (Traditional)

1 organic chicken (3–4 pounds), cut up with skin removed (or breast and leg meat with skin removed)
9 grams huang qi
4 pieces da zao
6 grams gan cao
6 grams shan yao
6 grams dang gui
organic chicken broth or water to cover

Combine all of the ingredients in a crock pot and cook on high for 1½–2 hours. Discard the herbs when the soup is ready.

Basic Beef Broth

2 pounds organic short ribs
1 pound organic beef marrow bones
3 quarts filtered water
1 large onion, quartered
1 fresh parsley sprig
1 carrot cut into small pieces
2 cabbage leaves
1 stalk celery cut into small pieces
5 peppercorns
1 teaspoon sea salt

In a large stock pot, combine the short ribs, beef bones, and water. Bring to a boil over high heat for 15 minutes, skimming often. Add the remaining ingredients and bring to a boil once again. Reduce heat and simmer for about 1½ hours, or until the meat is tender. Strain the broth (discarding bones, but keeping the meat for other dishes). Chill the broth until the fat separates from the liquid. Skim the fat. The broth stays fresh in the refrigerator for 2 days or can be frozen for future use.

Protein Shake

2 cups unsweetened organic soy milk
½ banana
1 teaspoon wheat germ
1 teaspoon almond powder

Combine all of the ingredients in a blender. Blend until smooth.

Black Sesame Oil Chicken Soup

¼ ounce fresh ginger root

4 tablespoons black sesame oil

4 pieces of halved organic chicken leg (have the butcher chop the
    chicken horizontally in half)

pinch of salt

1 bottle rice wine

*With a mallet or the flat side of a butcher knife, pound the ginger root
until it flattens, exposing the soft, fleshy part inside the root.*

*Pour the black sesame oil into a heated stainless steel pot. Swirl the oil
around the pot to cover the bottom and heat for about 15–20 seconds. Add
the ginger and stir it around for about 10–15 seconds. Add the chicken and
the salt. Stir-fry until the chicken is half cooked. Pour the rice wine into the
pot until it covers the chicken. Reduce heat to medium-low, cover, and continue to cook about 1 hour or until the chicken is done. Pour the broth and
a few pieces of chicken over brown rice or rice noodles and enjoy.*

Drunken Shrimp

2 cups filtered water

1 pound medium shrimp with shells

¼ ounce fresh ginger root

1 stalk green onion

3 cloves garlic

¼ cup rice wine

2 tablespoons sesame oil

pinch of salt

*In a saucepan, bring the water to a boil. Place the shrimp in the boiling wa-
ter and cook until the shrimp curl. Drain and run cold water over the shrimp.
Place the shrimp in a bowl and pat dry, then set aside to cool for about 15–
20 minutes. In the meantime, peel and slice the ginger, chop the green*

onion, and smash the garlic with the flat side of a knife. After the shrimp have cooled, pour the rice wine over them. Mix in the ginger, green onion, garlic, sesame oil, and add salt to taste. Marinate at room temperature for 1 hour.

The Chinese cook the shrimp, shell and all. This helps retain nutrients and flavor. The time to de-shell and de-vein is after cooking, while eating. Enjoy the shrimp over any whole-grain pasta and steamed snow peas.

Tonic Cereal

10 grams (about 2 sticks) Radix Codonopsis Pilosulae (dang sheng)
10 grams (about 2 sticks) Radix Astragali (huang qi)
5 cups filtered water
¼ cup Arillus Longanae (long yuan rou—longan fruit)
2 cups brown rice

Place the Codonopsis and Astragali in a nonmetallic container with the water and bring to a boil. Reduce the heat to low and cook for 30 minutes. Strain the liquid into a large bowl. Add the longan fruit and the rice, and steam over medium heat for 2 hours. A little honey may be added at the end.

Black Bean/Brown Rice Cereal

¼ cup black beans
4 cups filtered water
½ cup semen euryales (fox nut barley)
10 pieces Radix Dioscorreae (Chinese yam)
½ cup brown rice

Soak the black beans in the water overnight. Once soaked, place the beans, the barley, the Chinese yam, and the water in a blender, blend well, then pour into a large saucepan. Add the rice and steam for 1½–2 hours.

Herbal Chicken or Lamb Soup

3–4 pounds organic chicken (cut up, skin off) or 1½ pounds lamb
(for stew)

Herbal ingredients:

    Codonopsis (dang sheng): 10 grams—about 2–3 pieces

    Atractylodis (bai zhu): 9 grams

    Poriae (fu ling): 9 grams

    Honey-fried glycyrrhizae (zhi gan cao): 6 grams

    Rehmanniae (shu di): 9 grams

    Paeoniae (bai shao): 6 grams

    Angelica (dang gui): 9 grams

    Astragalus (huang qi): 10 grams

    Cinnamon twig (gui zhi): 3 grams

Combine all of the ingredients in a crock pot. Stew with 8 cups of filtered water for 3–4 hours. Discard the herbs before eating. Serve over whole grains of any kind.

Patient Fertility Questionnaire

Thank you for taking your valuable time to carefully complete this questionnaire. The information you provide will greatly help us in diagnosing, treating, and consulting with you regarding your condition.

Today's Date: _____ Date of Birth: _____ Age: _____ Ethnicity: _____

Name: _____

Your OB/GYN or Primary Physician: _____

Home Address: _____ City: _____

State: _____ Zip Code: _____ Home Phone: _____

Work Phone: _____ Email: _____

Fax: _____ Height: _____ Weight: _____

Occupation: _____ Marital Status: _____

Do you have a family history of the following conditions?
(Please check all that apply.)

☐ Autoimmune diseases ☐ Obesity ☐ DES usage

☐ Thyroid conditions ☐ Breast cancers ☐ Ovarian cancers

☐ Alcoholism ☐ Osteoporosis ☐ Other cancers

☐ Fertility issues ☐ Diabetes

Have you ever had or experienced any of the following conditions, even if it is resolved now? (Please check all that apply.)

☐ Anemia ☐ Fibromyalgia ☐ Anxiety

☐ Arthritis ☐ Lupus ☐ Sexually transmitted disease

☐ Abnormal pap smears ☐ Chronic fatigue ☐ Herpes genitalia

☐ Hearing impairment ☐ Endometriosis ☐ Bladder infection

☐ Visual impairment	☐ Ovarian cysts	☐ Uterine fibroids
☐ Urinary incontinence	☐ Digestive problems	☐ Elevated cholesterol
☐ Interstitial cystitis	☐ Constipation	☐ Skin cancer
☐ Cancer	☐ Diarrhea	☐ Heart disease
☐ Kidney infection	☐ Hemorrhoids	☐ Other cancers
☐ Heart disease	☐ Painful intercourse	☐ Diabetes mellitus
☐ Vaginal infection	☐ High blood pressure	☐ Thyroid disease
	☐ Diabetes	☐ Tuberculosis
☐ Kidney stones	☐ HIV/AIDS	☐ Pelvic inflammatory disease
☐ Sexually transmitted diseases	☐ Hepatitis	☐ Osteoporosis
☐ Autoimmune diseases	☐ Abdominal adhesions	☐ Liver disease
☐ Uterine polyps	☐ Abdominal or pelvic pains	☐ Gall stones
☐ Neurological disease	☐ Allergies/ sinusitis/skin conditions	☐ Fibroids
☐ Headaches	☐ Depression	☐ Polyps

	Never	Occasionally	Moderately	Frequently
Have you ever smoked?	☐	☐	☐	☐
Have you ever used alcohol?	☐	☐	☐	☐
Have you ever used caffeine?	☐	☐	☐	☐
Have you ever used marijuana?	☐	☐	☐	☐
Have you ever used recreational drugs?	☐	☐	☐	☐
Do you exercise regularly?	☐	☐	☐	☐

What age did you begin to menstruate? ☐ <11 ☐ 11 ☐ 12–14 ☐ 15 ☐ >15

Is your menstrual cycle regular? ☐ Yes ☐ No

What is the duration of your menstrual flow? ☐ <3 days ☐ 3–6 days ☐ >6 days

How is your overall menstrual flow? ☐ Light ☐ Moderate ☐ Heavy

How is your clotting during menstruation? ☐ None ☐ Few/Moderate ☐ Heavy

How would you rate the size of your clots? ☐ Small ☐ Medium ☐ Large

How are your menstrual cramps? ☐ None ☐ Medium/Moderate ☐ Severe

How long do your cramps last? ☐ Hours ☐ Days

Where are your menstrual cramps? (Check all that apply)

☐ None ☐ Pelvic ☐ Rectovaginal area
☐ Lower back ☐ Referring down the thighs/legs

Do you have irregular bleeding outside of your menstruation? ☐ Yes ☐ No

What are the symptoms you experience during ovulation? (Check all that apply.)

☐ None ☐ Vaginal discharge ☐ Increased libido
☐ Pelvic twinge ☐ Pelvic pain

Do you experience the following symptoms premenstrually? (Please check all that apply.)

☐ Anxiety ☐ Mood fluctuations ☐ Nervousness
☐ Fluid retention ☐ Food cravings ☐ Difficulty sleeping
☐ Headache ☐ Breast tenderness ☐ Constipation or bowel irregularity

How many total pregnancies? ☐ None ☐ 1 ☐ 2 ☐ 3 ☐ 4 or more

How many pregnancies carried to term? ☐ None ☐ 1 ☐ 2 ☐ 3 ☐ 4 or more

How many preterm
pregnancies? ☐ None ☐ 1 ☐ 2 ☐ 3 ☐ 4 or more

How many abortions? ☐ None ☐ 1 ☐ 2 ☐ 3 ☐ 4 or more

How many miscarriages? ☐ None ☐ 1 ☐ 2 ☐ 3 ☐ 4 or more

How many living
children? ☐ None ☐ 1 ☐ 2 ☐ 3 ☐ 4 or more

How old are they? ____ ____ ____ ____

	Yes	No
Do you have a history of sexual abuse or assault?	☐	☐
Are you satisfied with your sexual activities?	☐	☐
Do you have difficulties reaching orgasm?	☐	☐
Are you well lubricated during sexual intercourse?	☐	☐
Do you experience pain during sexual penetration?	☐	☐

What kind of contraception method have you used? (Check all that apply.)

☐ Oral contraceptives ☐ IUD ☐ Condom

☐ Sponges ☐ Diaphragm ☐ Withdrawal

☐ Rhythm ☐ Spermicidal gel

Have you encountered any difficulties with
your birth-control methods? ☐ Yes ☐ No

Have you had the following procedures/tests?

☐ 2nd- or 3rd-day serum ☐ Pregnancy termination
FSH/E2/Prolactin test ☐ Pelvic/Abdominal ultrasound

☐ Hysterosalpingography ☐ Mammography

☐ Hysteroscopy ☐ Laparoscopy

☐ Cervical conization ☐ Dilation and curettage

Please list all gynecological surgeries or procedures performed since birth:

Surgery *Age*

_____ _____

_____ _____

_____ _____

_____   _____
_____   _____
_____   _____
_____   _____
_____   _____

Please list all other surgeries or procedures performed since birth:

Surgery	Age

Has your partner
   had semen analysis?   ☐ Yes   ☐ No
What were the results?   ☐ Not applicable   ☐ Abnormal
   ☐ Normal
Do you have the following   ☐ Cat   ☐ Dog
   pets at home?   ☐ Rabbit   ☐ Others

Have you had the following procedures? (Please check that all apply.)
☐ Stimulated cycle without IUI   ☐ Stimulated IUI
☐ Non-stimulated IUI   ☐ GIFT
☐ ZIFT   ☐ IVF-FET
☐ IVF-DET

Basal Temperature Chart

Name: _____

Dates covered: ___/___/___ to ___/___/___

Cycle Day	1	2	3	4	5	6	7	8	9	10	11	12	13	14	15	16	17	18	19	20	21	22	23	24	25	26	27	28	29	30	31	32	33	34	35	36	37	38	39	40	41	42	43	44	45
Date																																													
Time																																													
99.0																																													
98.9																																													
98.8																																													
98.7																																													
98.6																																													
98.5																																													
98.4																																													
98.3																																													
98.2																																													
98.1																																													
98.0																																													
97.9																																													
97.8																																													
97.7																																													
97.6																																													
97.5																																													
97.4																																													
97.3																																													
97.2																																													
97.1																																													
97.0																																													
96.9																																													
96.8																																													
96.7																																													
96.6																																													
96.5																																													
Cervical Mucus																																													
Period																																													
Intercourse																																													
Cervical Mucus Textures																																													

RESOURCES

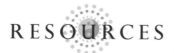

Couples and families with infertility need assistance coping with the emotional and practical aspects of this condition. For a more complete listing of infertility resources, go to www.taoofwellness.com/infertilityresources.

General Information and Support

American Society of Reproductive Medicine (ASRM)
205-978-5000
www.asrm.org

ASRM is a voluntary, nonprofit organization devoted to advancing knowledge and expertise in reproductive medicine, including infertility, menopause, contraception, and sexuality. This professional organization provides a wealth of information for both the public and professionals. The website also contains an area through the Society of Assisted Reproductive Technology (SART) that offers specific outcomes data from more than 347 infertility clinics around the United States. The SART database is the most up-to-date and user-friendly source of information on ART in the world.

National Institute of Child Health and Human Development (NICHD) Information Resource Center (IRC), National Institutes of Health
800-370-2943
http://www.nichd.nih.gov/health/topics/infertility_fertility.cfm

The NICHD Information Resource Center (IRC) provides information to the public on health issues within the NICHD research domain. By contacting the IRC, you'll have access to trained information specialists, health information, support organizations, and publication ordering. The website on infertility/fertility also lists NICHD-related clinical trials.

InterNational Council on Infertility Information Dissemination (INCIID)
703-379-9178
www.inciid.org

The InterNational Council on Infertility Information Dissemination (INCIID—pronounced "inside") is a nonprofit organization that helps individuals and couples explore their family-building options. INCIID provides current information and immediate support regarding the diagnosis, treatment, and prevention of infertility and pregnancy loss, and offers guidance to those considering adoption or a child-free lifestyle.

National Women's Health Information Center (NWHIC), U.S. Department of Health and Human Services
800-994-9662
http://womenshealth.gov/faq/infertility.htm

The National Women's Health Information Center (NWHIC) provides reliable and current information on women's health through a service of the Office on Women's Health (OWH) in the U.S. Department of Health and Human Services (HHS). There are more than eight hundred topics through the call center and website.

Office of Women's Health (OWH), U.S. Food and Drug Administration
888-INFO-FDA (888-463-6332)
http://www.fda.gov/womens/getthefacts/infertility.html

The U.S. Food and Drug Administration's Office of Women's Health (OWH) provides an overview on general infertility and medications used in infertility treatments.

Mayo Foundation for Medical Education and Research
800-446-2279

http://www.mayoclinic.com/health/infertility/DS00310

The Mayo Clinic is a not-for-profit medical practice dedicated to the diagnosis and treatment of virtually every type of complex illness. The website provides an overview of infertility conditions including a section on coping skills.

American Urological Association and Foundation
866-RING AUA (866-746-4282) or 410-689-3700

http://www.urologyhealth.org/adult/index.cfm?cat−11&topic=129

The American Urological Association and its foundation partner with physicians, researchers, health care professionals, patients, caregivers, families, and the public to support and promote research, patient/public education, and advocacy to improve the prevention, detection, treatment, and cure of urologic diseases. The website contains overview information on male infertility.

MedlinePlus, a Service of the U.S. National Library of Medicine (NLM) and the National Institutes of Health (NIH)
888-FINDNLM (888-346-3656) or 301-594-5983

http://www.nlm.nih.gov/medlineplus/infertility.html

#fromthenationalinstitutesofhealth

MedlinePlus, a web-based service, provides information and links to general and specific health topics. MedlinePlus brings together authoritative information from the NLM, the NIH, and other government agencies and health-related organizations. Searches in MedlinePlus give easy access to medical journal articles, drug information, an illustrated medical encyclopedia, interactive patient tutorials, and the latest health news. Specific and general information on infertility can be accessed through the link.

American College of Obstetricians and Gynecologists (ACOG)
Resource Center
202-638-5577
www.acog.org

The American College of Obstetricians and Gynecologists (ACOG), based in Washington, D.C., is a private, voluntary, nonprofit membership organization. It was founded in 1951 in Chicago and currently has more than forty-nine thousand members. It is the nation's leading group of professionals providing health care for women. Its website has minimal information for the general public on infertility, but it does have a section detailing publications on infertility-related issues.

RESOLVE: The National Infertility Association
301-652-8585
www.resolve.org

RESOLVE: The National Infertility Association, established in 1974, is a patient-driven nonprofit organization with the only established nationwide network of chapters mandated to promote reproductive health and to ensure equal access to all family-building options for men and women experiencing infertility or other reproductive disorders. It provides support services through its network of volunteers, members, and professionals for people with infertility and related issues.

American Fertility Association (AFA)
888-917-3777
www.theafa.org

The American Fertility Association (AFA), a national nonprofit organization headquartered in New York City, was founded in 1999. The AFA provides a range of services designed to help people gather information about medical treatments, options, coping techniques, legal and insurance issues, and other concerns.

World Health Organization (WHO), United Nations (UN)
(+ 41 22) 791 21 11, Geneva, Switzerland
http://www.who.int/topics/infertility/en/

The World Health Organization is the United Nations' specialized agency for health. It was established on April 7, 1948. The website contains its publications, though a limited amount of information on infertility.

Acupuncture and Traditional Chinese Medicine

Tao of Wellness Clinics
310-917-2200
www.taoofwellness.com

Tao of Wellness clinics provide traditional Chinese medicine and acupuncture medical services for infertility and other general and specific conditions. It is the home clinic of the author. The website provides general and specific information on infertility as well as tools and contact information.

IVF Acupuncture Services (IAS)
888-IVF-0011
www.ivfacupuncture.com

IVF Acupuncture Services (IAS) was created to assist IVF clinics in providing the highest-quality, evidence-based acupuncture services for their patients. The creation of IAS came about from the lack of standardization and specialization bodies in the field of acupuncture in the United States. The author is a founding member of this organization. The website also contains the latest research information on acupuncture and IVF.

Acupuncture.com
www.acupuncture.com

The premier site on information relating to traditional Chinese medicine and acupuncture has a section to help patients find acupuncturists in their locale.

American Board of Oriental Reproductive Medicine
www.aborm.org

This board was formed by leading professionals in oriental reproductive medicine who come together with a resolve to set the standard of care in this field. It provides a certification process to practitioners who are treating patients with oriental medicine in the field of reproductive health. A section of the website devoted to a list of board-certified professionals is currently undergoing development.

National Certification Commission for Acupuncture and Oriental Medicine (NCCAOM)
904-598-1005
www.nccaom.org

The National Certification Commission for Acupuncture and Oriental Medicine (NCCAOM) is a nonprofit organization established in 1982. Its mission is to establish, assess, and promote recognized standards of competence and safety in acupuncture and oriental medicine for the protection and benefit of the public. It provides a searchable database of its diplomates in acupuncture.

Polycystic Ovarian Syndrome

Polycystic Ovarian Syndrome Association (PCOSA)
www.pcosupport.org

PCOSA is a national nonprofit organization dedicating its advocacy, service, and support to the patients of polycystic ovarian syndrome. It is located in Englewood, Colorado, and its website has links and information on issues relating to polycystic ovarian disease.

Endometriosis

Endometriosis Association
800-992-3636 or 414-355-2200
www.endometriosisassn.org

The Endometriosis Association was the first organization in the world created for those with endometriosis. As an independent self-help non-profit organization of women with endometriosis, doctors, and others interested in the disease, it is a recognized authority in its field whose goal is to work toward finding a cure for the disease as well as to provide education, support, and research.

Endometriosis.org
www.endometriosis.org

Endometriosis.org strives to be the global platform for news and information on endometriosis. It facilitates collaboration and information sharing between women with endometriosis, physicians, scientists, and others interested in the disease. Endometriosis.org is a nonprofit organization.

Cancer and Infertility

American Cancer Society
800-ACS-2345 (800-227-2345)
http://www.cancer.org/docroot/MBC/MBC_2x_Fertility_and_
Cancer.asp?sitearea=&level=

The American Cancer Society is a nationwide community-based volunteer health organization dedicated to eliminating cancer as a major health problem by preventing cancer, saving lives, and diminishing suffering from cancer, through research, education, advocacy, and service. The website provides general information on infertility as well as information for cancer patients whose medical treatments present the risk of infertility.

Fertile Hope
888-994-4673
www.fertilehope.org

Fertile Hope is a nationwide nonprofit organization dedicated to providing reproductive information, support, and hope to cancer patients whose medical treatments present the risk of infertility. Fertile Hope is partnered with the Lance Armstrong Foundation to help meet the profound needs of patients whose medical treatments present the risk of infertility. The organization was founded in 2001 by cancer survivor Lindsay Nohr Beck as a result of her own endeavors to preserve her fertility in the face of critical cancer treatments. Fertile Hope is headquartered in New York City.

Adoption and Pregnancy

Child Welfare Information Gateway, Children's Bureau, U.S. Department of Health and Human Services
800-394-3366 or 703-385-7565
http://www.childwelfare.gov/pubs/f_adoptoptionglance.cfm

Child Welfare Information Gateway promotes the safety, permanency, and well-being of children and families by connecting child welfare, adoption, and related professionals as well as concerned citizens to timely, essential information. This link provides an overview of the adoption process. It also contains a U.S. National Adoption Directory with state-by-state contact information for a variety of adoption-related organizations and services including public and licensed private adoption agencies, support groups, state reunion registries, and more.

American Pregnancy Association
800-672-2296
www.americanpregnancy.org

The American Pregnancy Association is a nonprofit national health organization committed to promoting reproductive and pregnancy wellness
through education, research, advocacy, and community awareness. The
association has an adoption directory referral service as well as general and
specific information on the adoption process.

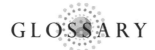

GLOSSARY

acidophilus: a type of bacteria that grows in our intestines. It assists in containing yeast growth and provides a healthy digestive environment for the intestines.

acupuncture: a therapy that involves inserting, retaining, and manipulating one or a group of thin needles into different areas of the body to solicit therapeutic response.

adenomyosis: a condition where endometrial tissue grows inside the myometrium, the muscular layer of the uterus.

antiphospholipid syndrome: also called Hughes syndrome. This is a condition where the patient is prone to clotting, especially during pregnancy, increasing the risk of miscarriage.

BBT: basal body temperature. It is the body temperature at rest without any movement or food intake. It is taken orally each morning immediately upon waking. Recording these temperatures on a chart helps to study the rise and fall of hormones and offers a retrospective prediction of probable ovulation time.

blood stagnation: a disorder pattern in traditional Chinese medicine. It points to pain and cardiovascular disorders.

BMI: body mass index. It is a measure of body fat based on height and weight that applies to both adult men and women.

Buddha: an enlightened spiritual being in Buddhism, a religion of India. A Buddha is a spiritual being that has overcome desire, craving, aversion, and delusion and has attained complete liberation from suffering.

cerclage: a procedure where the cervix is sewn up to prevent miscarriage.

chi: see **qi.**

chi gong: see **qi gong.**

chlamydia: a type of vaginal bacterial infection, frequently asymptomatic, that will affect fertility if left untreated.

Clomid: clomiphene citrate. It is a fertility drug that promotes multiple egg development and is frequently the first-line drug used in treating infertility conditions.

clomiphene citrate challenge test (CCCT): a test where an analysis of follicle-stimulating hormone (FSH) is taken before and after a period of Clomid usage in the stimulation of ovaries to measure relative ovarian reserve.

C-section: cesarean section. Surgical delivery of the baby by incision of the abdominal and uterine wall.

D&C: dilation and curettage. A frequently performed procedure during miscarriage to remove any remaining conception products in the uterus, it involves dilation of the cervix and scraping of the uterine lining.

dermoid cyst: a nonmalignant cyst in the ovary that contains epidermal skin cells capable of developing into nails, hairs, and teeth in the ovary.

DES: diethylstilbesterol. A form of synthetic estrogen formerly used to prevent miscarriages in women in the 1950s and 1960s. It has been implicated in birth defects of the reproductive tract in the offspring of women who took DES during pregnancy.

diabetes mellitus: a condition of dysfunction of sugar metabolism in the body.

Eight Treasures: a group of meditative exercises that have been passed down through generations in the Ni family. It combines breathing, focus, imagery, stretching, holding, and strength to invigorate your qi, blood, and overall vitality.

electroacupuncture: a type of acupuncture using a small electrostimulator that sends a small amount of microampere or milliampere electrical current through acupuncture needles to the affected area to enhance therapeutic effects.

embryo: a fertilized egg. In human reproduction, this is the earliest stage of the fertilization of the egg and the sperm.

endometriosis: a condition where endometrial tissue grows outside of the uterus.

endometrium: the blood- and nutrient-rich tissue that lines the inside of the uterus. It grows and sheds with each menstrual cycle.

endorphins: hormone-like protein substances secreted by the brain. Endorphins regulate our mood and manage our perception of pain.

epidural: administered during labor to reduce pain by injecting anesthesia into spinal spaces in the lower back region.

estrogen: a hormone secreted primarily in the ovaries and in small amounts in the testes. It has an array of functions that include stimulation of female secondary sex characteristics, stimulation of ovulation, induction of menstruation, maintenance of normal nervous system activity, bone density, and pregnancy.

fallopian tubes: a pair of tubes that connect the ovaries to the uterus. This is where fertilization normally takes place; that is, where the egg from the ovary meets the sperm.

feng shui: directly translated as "wind and water." Originally a study of geography and how it affects human lives, nowadays it is used to describe a study of how the placement of objects in a living space or work space affects our life.

five tastes: a basic grouping of major tastes used in the traditional Chinese medicine diagnosis of diseases and classification of herbs and foods. It consists of sour, bitter, sweet, pungent, and salty.

four qualities: used to describe the nature of foods and herbs in traditional Chinese medicine. They consist of cold, cool, warm, and hot.

FSH: follicle-stimulating hormone. It is a hormone secreted by the anterior pituitary gland in the brain and is responsible for egg stimulation and growth in the ovaries.

HELLP: an acronym or syndrome of hemolysis (a breakdown of red blood cells), elevated liver enzyme levels, and low platelets during the late stages of pregnancy. It is a form of severe toxemia/preeclampsia. See also **preeclampsia; toxemia.**

HSG: hysterosalpingography. It is a testing procedure involving X-ray that uses dye to visualize the patency (openness) of the fallopian tubes.

hydrosalpinx: a condition where the fallopian tube is dilated and filled with fluid.

hyperthyroid: a condition where the thyroid gland produces and secretes abnormally high levels of the thyroid hormone thyroxin.

hypothyroid: a condition where the thyroid gland produces and secretes abnormally low levels of the thyroid hormone thyroxin.

hysteroscopy: a diagnostic procedure using a lighted scope to examine the inside of the uterus. It is a commonly utilized procedure in infertility when there is suspicion of fibroids, polyps, septa, adhesions, or any other abnormalities of the uterus.

God of Heaven: a spiritual being that governs Heaven in Chinese mythology and religions.

IVF: in vitro fertilization. A procedure where the eggs from a woman are retrieved from the ovaries, fertilized in a laboratory dish with sperm, and transferred back to the uterus.

IVIG: intravenous immune globulin. Globulin is sterile protein derived from human blood. IVIG is used in cases of immunological infertility condition to reduce rejection of pregnancy by the mother's body.

kidney yang deficiency: a disorder pattern in traditional Chinese medicine. It points to weakness in the endocrine, cardiovascular, and metabolic systems.

kidney yin deficiency: a disorder pattern in traditional Chinese medicine. It points to weakness in the endocrine, genitourinary, and reproductive systems.

Lao Tzu: a Chinese philosopher in the sixth century B.C. known for his establishment of the philosophy of Tao and his work, *Dao De Jin,* which exerted great influence on traditional Chinese medicine and Chinese culture.

LH: luteinizing hormone. It is a hormone secreted by the anterior pituitary gland in the brain and is responsible for egg maturation and release from the ovary.

liver qi stasis: a disorder pattern in traditional Chinese medicine. It points to imbalances in hepatic, nervous, and endocrine systems.

lupus: a systemic autoimmune disease that attacks different tissues of the body.

luteal phase defect: a shortened luteal phase. A luteal phase lasts approximately fourteen days from ovulation to the onset of menstruation. A luteal phase of less than ten to twelve days is considered to be a luteal phase defect.

Mandarin: originally a dialect spoken in northern China. It has been standardized as the national language for all of China.

meridian: a pathway on our body that consists of different acupuncture points. In acupuncture, there are twelve main meridians that run throughout the body. These meridians are connected with associated organs and are used to diagnose and treat dysfunctions of these organs.

microsystem: a system of imaging of the entire body from a small part of the body for our purpose of diagnosis and treatment. For example, in the ear microsystem, various parts of the ear correspond to different parts of the body. By treating and palpating certain parts of the ear, imbalances in certain parts of the body can be detected.

Monkey King: named Sun Wu Kong, a mythical humanized monkey figure. He is the main character in the book *The Journey to the West* written by Cheng En Wu in A.D. 1500. He symbolizes strength, character, righteousness, and defiance. The book is a classic for Chinese readers.

mycoplasma: a type of bacterial infection that attacks the genitourinary tract and the lung. It has been implicated in miscarriages.

patterns: a method for how traditional Chinese medicine practitioners diagnose diseases by grouping collections of symptoms and signs.

perimenopause: a transitional period of time just before menopause in which a woman experiences perceptible physiological changes and symptoms.

phlegm-damp congestion: a disorder pattern in traditional Chinese medicine. It points to possible gastrointestinal, immunological, infectious, and oncological disorders.

Pin Yin: also known as Hanyu Pin Yin. It is the most common Mandarin romanization used today. Roman letters are used to represent the phonetic translation of Mandarin sounds.

PCOS: polycystic ovarian syndrome. It is a condition characterized by irregular or missed periods, elevated androgen (male hormone) levels, and polycystic structures in the ovaries visualized by ultrasound.

preeclampsia: a toxic condition usually occurring in the late stages of pregnancy with symptoms of high blood pressure, swelling, and protein in the urine.

PRL: prolactin. It is a hormone secreted by the anterior pituitary gland in the brain and is responsible for breast and breast milk development.

probiotics: a dietary supplement. It contains a variety of beneficial bacteria and yeasts that promote better intestinal health and digestion.

progesterone: a female sex hormone. Secreted by the ovaries after ovulation, it prepares the uterine lining for implantation.

pulse diagnosis: a distinct method of traditional Chinese medicine for diagnosing disease conditions by evaluating the pulse, usually the radial pulse in the wrist area.

qi: a direct phonetic translation from Chinese. It means energy. In general, it is used to describe energy in the universe. Specifically, it describes energy in the body, especially energy that runs through the meridians, organ systems, and all corners of the body.

qi gong: a therapeutic and healthy meditative exercise combining specific breathing techniques, guided imagery, and movements to improve health and treat disease.

rheumatoid arthritis: an autoimmune condition in which the body's immune system attacks the joints.

sonohysterogram: a type of ultrasound of the uterus involving the injection of saline solution into the uterine cavity for better visualization while checking for abnormal structures such as polyps or fibroids.

syndromes: a collection of symptoms and signs that denotes a particular type of condition or disease.

Tai Ji: a principle of infinity from which all things in the cosmos evolve. It is the principle that precedes the differentiation and existence of yin and yang.

tai chi chuan: or tai ji quan. It is an internal martial arts practice that originated in 1820 consisting of a group of continuous flowing movements used for self-defense and meditation.

Taiwan: Formosa, "beautiful island" in Portuguese. It is located in East Asia off the coast of mainland China. It consists of steep mountains covered by tropical and subtropical vegetation sharing the same latitude as the Hawaiian islands and similar climate patterns.

Tao: a philosophy, methodology, and system of knowledge that contemplates the workings of the universe, nature, and the relationship of humankind in the world.

TCM: traditional Chinese medicine. A comprehensive system of health care knowledge that has been practiced in China for centuries and has now spread to many different parts of the world.

tongue diagnosis: a distinct method of traditional Chinese medicine that diagnoses a disease condition by evaluating the tongue.

toxemia: pregnancy-induced hypertension that can endanger the health of the baby and the mother.

TSH: thyroid-stimulating hormone. It is a hormone secreted by the anterior pituitary gland that regulates the function of the thyroid gland, which influences metabolism, growth, and development, and can affect reproductive functions.

ultrasound: ultrasonography. It is a procedure using high-energy sound waves to create an image of the body's internal organs and structures.

ureaplasma: a type of bacterial infection that frequently attacks the genitourinary tract, causing inflammation in the pelvis in women and in the prostate in men.

UTI: urinary tract infection. Microorganisms such as bacteria can invade the urinary tract to cause infection and inflammation.

yin: part of a dichotomy concept, with yang, rooted deeply in the Chinese culture, philosophy, and medicine. It denotes the feminine, softer, gentler, passive side of nature.

yang: part of a dichotomy concept, with yin, rooted deeply in the Chinese culture, philosophy, and medicine. It denotes the masculine, harder, rougher, active side of nature.

INDEX